ADOLESCENT PSYCHOTHERAPY

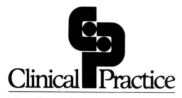

Clinical Practice

Number 16

Judith H. Gold, M.D., F.R.C.P.(C)
Series Editor

ADOLESCENT PSYCHOTHERAPY

Edited by

Marcia Slomowitz, M.D.

Associate Professor of Clinical Psychiatry
Director of Medical Student Education
Associate Director of Residency Training
College of Medicine
University of Cincinnati
Cincinnati, Ohio

Washington, DC
London, England

Copyright © 1991 American Psychiatric Press, Inc.
ALL RIGHTS RESERVED
Manufactured in the United States of America on acid-free paper. ∞
93 92 91 90 4 3 2 1

American Psychiatric Press, Inc.
1400 K St., N.W., Washington, DC 20005

Library of Congress Cataloging-in-Publication Data

Adolescent psychotherapy/edited by Marcia Slomowitz.
      p.   cm.—(Clinical practice ; no. 16)
    Includes bibliographical references.
    ISBN 0-88048-181-1 (alk. paper)
    1. Adolescent psychotherapy. I. Slomowitz, Marcia. 1949–
II. Series.
    [DNLM: 1. Psychotherapy—in adolescence. W1 CL767J no. 16/WS
463 A2397]
RJ503.A323   1990
616.89′14′0835—dc20
DNLM/DLC   90-871
for Library of Congress   CIP

British Library Cataloguing in Publication Data

A CIP record is available from the British Library.

Contents

Contributors

Seth Aronson, Psy.D.
Coordinator, Child-Adolescent Group Therapy, Bronx
Municipal Hospital Center—Albert Einstein College of
Medicine, Bronx, New York

Dewleen G. Baker, M.D.
Assistant Professor of Psychiatry, College of Medicine,
University of Cincinnati, Cincinnati, Ohio

Jules R. Bemporad, M.D.
Professor of Clinical Psychiatry, Cornell Medical College;
Director of Education, Westchester Division, Cornell Medical
Center, White Plains, New York

Robert M. Galatzer-Levy, M.D., S.C.
Lecturer in Psychiatry, University of Chicago; Faculty,
Chicago Institute for Psychoanalysis, Chicago, Illinois

Kathleen J. Hart, Ph.D.
Assistant Professor of Psychology, Xavier University,
Cincinnati, Ohio

Robert L. Hendren, D.O.
Associate Professor of Psychiatry and Pediatrics; Director,
Division of Child and Adolescent Psychiatry, University of
New Mexico Medical Center, Albuquerque, New Mexico

Charles M. Jaffe, M.D.
Assistant Professor of Psychiatry, Rush Medical College;
Lecturer, Department of Psychiatry and Behavioral Sciences,
Northwestern University Medical School; Faculty, Chicago
Institute for Psychoanalysis, Chicago, Illinois

Richard C. Marohn, M.D.
Professor of Clinical Psychiatry, Northwestern University
Medical School; Faculty, Chicago Institute for Psychoanalysis;
Private practice—psychiatry and psychoanalysis, Chicago,
Illinois

John E. Meeks, M.D.
Medical Director, Psychiatric Institute of Montgomery
County, Rockville, Maryland

Glen T. Pearson, Jr., M.D.
Clinical Associate Professor of Psychiatry, University of
Texas Southwestern Medical Center; Director, Adolescent
Boys' Unit, Timberlawn Psychiatric Hospital, Dallas, Texas

Saul Scheidlinger, Ph.D.
Professor of Psychiatry (Child Psychology), Albert Einstein
College of Medicine, Bronx, New York

Marcia Slomowitz, M.D.
Associate Professor of Clinical Psychiatry; Director of
Medical Student Education; Associate Director of Residency
Training, College of Medicine, University of Cincinnati,
Cincinnati, Ohio

Introduction
to the Clinical Practice Series

Over the years of its existence the series of monographs entitled *Clinical Insights* gradually became focused on providing current, factual, and theoretical material of interest to the clinician working outside of a hospital setting. To reflect this orientation, the name of the Series has been changed to *Clinical Practice*.

The Clinical Practice Series will provide readers with books that give the mental health clinician a practical clinical approach to a variety of psychiatric problems. These books will provide up-to-date literature reviews and emphasize the most recent treatment methods. Thus, the publications in the Series will interest clinicians working both in psychiatry and in the other mental health professions.

Each year a number of books will be published dealing with all aspects of clinical practice. In addition, from time to time when appropriate, the publications may be revised and updated. Thus, the Series will provide quick access to relevant and important areas of psychiatric practice. Some books in the Series will be authored by a person considered to be an expert in that particular area; others will be edited by such an expert who will also draw together other knowledgeable authors to produce a comprehensive overview of that topic.

Some of the books in the Clinical Practice Series will have their foundation in presentations at an annual meeting of the American Psychiatric Association. All will contain the most recently available information on the subjects discussed. Theoretical and scientific data will be applied to clinical situations, and case illustrations will be utilized in order to make the material even more relevant for the practitioner. Thus, the Clinical Practice Series should provide educational reading in a compact format especially written for the mental health clinician–psychiatrist.

Judith H. Gold, M.D., F.R.C.P.(C)
Series Editor
Clinical Practice Series

Clinical Practice Series Titles

Treating Chronically Mentally Ill Women (#1)
Edited by Leona L. Bachrach, Ph.D., and Carol C. Nadelson, M.D.

Divorce as a Developmental Process (#2)
Edited by Judith H. Gold, M.D., F.R.C.P.(C)

Family Violence: Emerging Issues of a National Crisis (#3)
Edited by Leah J. Dickstein, M.D., and Carol C. Nadelson, M.D.

Anxiety and Depressive Disorders in the Medical Patient (#4)
By Leonard R. Derogatis, Ph.D., and Thomas N. Wise, M.D.

Anxiety: New Findings for the Clinician (#5)
Edited by Peter Roy-Byrne, M.D.

The Neuroleptic Malignant Syndrome and Related Conditions (#6)
By Arthur Lazarus, M.D., Stephan C. Mann, M.D., and Stanley N. Caroff, M.D.

Juvenile Homicide (#7)
Edited by Elissa P. Benedek, M.D., and Dewey G. Cornell, Ph.D.

Measuring Mental Illness: Psychometric Assessment for Clinicians (#8)
Edited by Scott Wetzler, Ph.D.

Family Involvement in Treatment of the Frail Elderly (#9)
Edited by Marion Zucker Goldstein, M.D.

Psychiatric Care of Migrants: A Clinical Guide (#10)
By Joseph J. Westermeyer, M.D., M.P.H., Ph.D.

Office Treatment of Schizophrenia (#11)
Edited by Mary V. Seeman, M.D., F.R.C.P.(C), and Stanley E. Greben, M.D., F.R.C.P.(C)

The Psychosocial Impact of Job Loss (#12)
By Nick Kates, M.B.B.S., F.R.C.P.(C), Barrie S. Greiff, M.D., and Duane Q. Hagen, M.D.

New Perspectives on Narcissism (#13)
Edited by Eric M. Plakun, M.D.

Clinical Management of Gender Identity Disorders in Children and Adults (#14)
Edited by Ray Blanchard, Ph.D., and Betty W. Steiner, M.B., F.R.C.P.(C)

Family Approaches in Treatment of Eating Disorders (#15)
Edited by D. Blake Woodside, M.D., M.Sc., F.R.C.P.(C), and Lorie Shekter-Wolfson, M.S.W., C.S.W.

Adolescent Psychotherapy (#16)
Edited by Marcia Slomowitz, M.D.

Benzodiazepines in Clinical Practice: Risks and Benefits (#17)
Edited by Peter P. Roy-Byrne, M.D., and Deborah S. Cowley, M.D.

Current Treatments of Obsessive-Compulsive Disorder (#18)
Edited by Michele Tortora Pato, M.D., and Joseph Zohar, M.D.

Chapter 1

Introduction

MARCIA SLOMOWITZ, M.D.

Chapter 1

Introduction

Psychiatric morbidity is increasing for adolescents. The rates of depression are rising, as are the rates of suicide attempts and completions, alcoholism and drug use, and teen pregnancy (Holinger 1979; Klerman 1988; Miller 1982; Shaffer and Fisher 1981).

These events are occurring in a context of considerable social change. The divorce rate in the United States is approximately 50%, resulting in adolescents living in single-parent or blended families. Roles of women have changed, with an increased number of women in the work force. There is also greater geographical mobility. The instability of the surrounding social environment means that the most dependent, the children, are at risk for psychiatric distress (Klerman and Weissman 1989).

Only recently have longitudinal studies brought into focus the variety of responses and defense patterns enacted by children and adolescents who have experienced family disruption, divorce, and remarriage (Wallerstein and Blakeslee 1989). Interpersonal difficulties and depression are a consequence of these changes and may continue unremitting into adulthood (Kandel and Davies 1986). This phenomenon represents only one of a multitude of interactions between social forces and intrapsychic functioning.

Concomitantly, there has been an expansion of models for psychotherapeutic intervention. Older, rigidly applied treatment procedures have given way to greater treatment flexibility. Yet a firm foundation in understanding psychotherapy remains essential if a therapist is to integrate ideas from the various innovations and to assess which of these ideas are useful and which are not. All of this takes place against a backdrop of rapid advances in understanding biological factors impacting on and interacting with the adolescent and the family. The overall result is that psychotherapists working with adolescents have available a vastly increased fund of knowledge that can be usefully applied to their work.

Among other factors, the dramatic shortage of child and adolescent psychiatrists has created a situation in which the delivery of psychotherapeutic services is predominantly provided by other mental health professionals. The forecast is a need for 10,000 child psychiatrists by the 1990s, a goal that will not be attained in light of the current roster of approximately 5,000 (Crowley 1985; Philips et al. 1983). This book provides an important base for clinicians of all disciplines conducting psychotherapy with adolescents and their families.

Adolescent Psychotherapy has as its approach a biopsychosocial framework. This viewpoint allows us to appreciate more freely the advances in each of the three spheres, and affords an opportunity to reconceptualize the traditional dyadic relationship of treatment. Several models of psychotherapy are discussed, but no one approach is presented as the "best one."

The book is organized into three sections. The first section, Chapters 2–4, introduces each of the three components of the biopsychosocial framework. The second section, Chapters 5 and 6, details issues relevant to individual, family, and group psychotherapy with adolescents. The third section, Chapters 7–10, addresses the treatment of common disorders. These divisions have been made for heuristic purposes; they provide a map for the clinician. In practice the issues overlap, and therefore therapists may wish to consult a number of chapters to further refine and broaden their theoretical outlook.

The authors were chosen because of their interest and expertise in a specific area and recognition of the importance of integrating the biological, psychological, and social aspects of psychotherapy. All are active practitioners, and their extensive experiences in working with adolescents will be apparent.

Theory

Jaffe, in the second chapter, summarizes psychoanalytic theories of adolescence and provides an historical context for contemporary views. Beginning with Anna Freud on the intrinsic turmoil in adolescence, he moves to Blos's emphasis on the primacy of psychological change brought on by the sexual transfigurations of puberty, Masterson's discussion of the recapitulation of the separation-individuation phase of early childhood, and Kohut's centrality of the adolescent's transformation of ideals as a means of reorganizing the self. Citing findings from studies involving child and adolescent observation and clinical work, Jaffe critiques these theories and provides what he considers a more contemporary view, that of Michael Basch. Jaffe emphasizes the adolescent's push for competence and adaptation as prime psychological forces and thus asks the reader to consider psychotherapy as applied developmental psychology focused on the empathic mode of understanding the individual's subjective experience.

Biological and neurodevelopmental factors are the subject of Chapter 3 by Baker and Hart. The authors begin the chapter by discussing the adolescent with neurologically based learning disabilities. These developmental disabilities contribute to psychiatric morbidity, depression, and low self-esteem. The authors discuss the usefulness of various types of psychotherapies for such individuals in conjunction with educational intervention. They then discuss mood disorders in adolescence, whose existence has been controversial until the emergence of reliable and valid semistructured interviews. While the symptoms of depression are similar to those in adults, certain symptoms, such as hopelessness, helplessness, and hypersomnia, are more severe in adolescents than in adults. In addition, the depression itself is more severe when the mood disorder is accompanied by a conduct, learning, or attention-deficit disorder. Research into the efficacy of antidepressant medications is limited in comparison with that of adults and shows these medications to be useful in a smaller number of patients. A hypothesis for this finding is that alterations in brain physiology during adolescence result in changes in the pharmacodynamics of the tricyclic antidepressants.

The social context in which the adolescent lives is discussed by Pearson in Chapter 4. A social systems approach is used to conceptualize the roles and functions of the community, school, family, individual, and therapist. The dyad of patient-therapist is seldom insulated from the interface with the adolescent's other systems. It is the task of the therapist to articulate, monitor, and often regulate these boundaries. For instance, engagement of the family in psychotherapy for the purpose of improving their functioning is distinguished from involving family members, particularly parents, for gathering information or developing a contractual relationship. Pearson suggests that ethnic and racial vicissitudes be brought into the treatment, imploring us to not overlook the effects of racism on a child. Finally, he provides a practical approach to working with the school system, an often over-looked ally of the adolescent and therapist in our changing society.

Treatment

Galatzer-Levy, in Chapter 5, provides an overview of the psychotherapeutic process. Organized around psychoanalytic concepts, the chapter addresses the following critical issues: goals of psychotherapy, the working alliance with the teenager and family, transference and countertransference phenomena, and the termination process. From Galatzer-Levy's perspective, the general principles of psychotherapy with adolescents are not different from those used in working with adults. The major goal is to renew the capacity for growth and development of the individual. He notes that the therapist will find that work with this population has special qualities, characterized by variability and intensity of affects due to changes in the body, cognitive capacity, and image of the self, and also to changes in the reactivity of adolescents to environmental pressures.

The sixth chapter, by Scheidlinger and Aronson, focuses on group psychotherapy. Recognizing the importance of the peer group in adolescence for promoting self-esteem, social maturation, and emancipation from the family, these authors emphasize a group approach as the treatment of choice. The psychotherapy group becomes a vehicle for intrapsychic and interpersonal transformations. Indications for group therapy, either in conjunction with or as the sole modality of treatment, are given. The appropriateness of fit of the specific individual to a given group, problems associated with younger versus older adolescents, themes encountered, and therapeutic factors identified as helpful are also described.

Specific Disorders and Their Treatment

The final four chapters discuss psychotherapy of adolescents with specific disorders. Each author uses an integrative treatment approach.

Hendren begins this section with a discussion on attention-deficit disorder in Chapter 7. Biological factors such as the genetic propensity to acquire this disorder, psychological issues of low self-regard and characterological dilemmas, and accompanying social and academic problems are addressed. He argues for a multipronged approach to treatment with these individuals, and details use of medication, individualized educational interventions, and psychological work. Hendren notes that newer cognitive approaches may be instrumental in the treatment of these individuals. It is fitting that the initial chapter of this section integrates the biological, psychological, and social themes in a syndrome often neglected in the psychotherapy literature.

The psychotherapy of adolescents with behavioral disorders is discussed in Chapter 8 by Marohn. He asks us to consider understanding the meaning of the behavior for the individual and portrays treatment of individuals with these disorders with great sensitivity. For example, violent behavior may occur in an adolescent experiencing a traumatic overstimulation, feeling overwhelmed by strong wishes for affectionate contact. Some violent acts may be an attempt to destroy an offending other who has failed to live up to idealized expectations. Other behavior may be a turning of a narcissistic injury into an external assault in an attempt to reconstitute a crumbling self. Suicide is a possibility, as some adolescents may prefer to kill themselves than to become consciously aware that their parents may consider them expendable. In this context Marohn discusses the setting for treatment that may change depending on the need for external containment, as with inpatient and residential settings. He discusses the indications for psychopharmacological treatment as a component of the overall treatment plan.

In Chapter 9, Bemporad describes the psychotherapy of adolescents with unipolar and bipolar disorders. He categorizes unipolar depression into two types: an "anaclitic" depression whose roots entail a continuing symbiotic tie to a need-fulfilling parent, and an "introjective" depression in which the individual may have more successfully individualized from the parents but has internalized severe parental standards. In both forms, the adolescent's inner perceptions are of failure to cope with the psychosocial demands of growing up, resulting in profound despair. Support and reparenting, and acceptance of the individual's feelings of shame and failure, are both particularly poignant aspects of psychotherapy with these individuals.

Neurotic conflict may plague adolescents and is the subject explored by Meeks in the final chapter. These adolescents suffer severely from discomfort associated with self-blame and negative self-regard. The dysphoria is experienced as a combination of anxiety and/or depression. While the adolescent feels deficient, he or she has some awareness that these feelings have an irrational component. The diagnosis is predicated, as Meeks points out, on the patient's "magical use of the imagination" in an attempt to resolve this inner conflict. Rich vignettes are illustrative of such intrapsychic conflicts and the psychotherapeutic process.

In conclusion, this book has combined theory and practice in a man-

ner useful to clinicians working with adolescents in the 1990s. The authors have brought together the most recent theoretical and empirical advances with actual clinical experience to make this an engrossing book.
Their sensitive concern for their patients' lives and dilemmas enriches
the text. These authors' contributions are helpful in understanding and
working with the individual casualties of ever greater societal changes.
Continuing modifications of psychoanalytic theory moving toward a
more empathic and adaptive view of adolescence, fundamental discoveries from biological research, and appreciation for the social systems
changes affecting modern treatment will contribute to the future directions of adolescent psychotherapy.

References

Crowley AE: Graduate Medical Education in the United States, 1984–1985.
    JAMA 254:1585–1593, 1985

Holinger PC: Violent deaths among the young: recent trends in suicide, homi-
    cide, and accidents. Am J Psychiatry 136:1144–1147, 1979

Kandel DB, Davies G: Adult sequelae of adolescent depressive symptoms.
    Arch Gen Psychiatry 43:255–264, 1986

Klerman GL: The current age of youthful melancholia: evidence for increase
    in depression among adolescents and young adults. Br J Psychiatry 152:
    4–14, 1988

Klerman GL, Weissman MM: Increasing rates of depression. JAMA 261:
    2229–2235, 1989

Miller J: National survey on drug abuse: main findings (DHHS Publ No 83-
    1263). Washington, DC, U.S. Government Printing Office, 1982

Philips J, Cohen RZ, Enzer WB: Child Psychiatry: A Plan for the Coming
    Decades. Washington, DC, American Academy of Child Psychiatry, 1983

Shaffer D, Fisher P: The epidemiology of suicide in children and young ad-
    olescents. J Am Acad Child Psychiatry 20:545–565, 1981

Wallerstein JS, Blakeslee SH: Second Chances: Men, Women, and Children a
    Decade After Divorce. New York, Ticknor and Fields, 1989

Theory

Chapter 2

Psychology: Psychoanalytic Approaches to Adolescent Development

CHARLES M. JAFFE, M.D.

Chapter 2

Psychology: Psychoanalytic Approaches to Adolescent Development

Psychotherapy with adolescents has long been recognized as particularly challenging because these young people come for help with specific problems in adaptation while they are in the midst of rapid developmental change. Anna Freud (1958) noted the difficulty understanding adolescents because of the many polarities evident in their behavior. The rapid fluctuation and range of behaviors typical of the period can make diagnosis and treatment difficult. It may be hard to understand adolescents because their modes of expression are often action oriented and engender strong responses in those around them. In addition, adolescents are often elusive with the adults who become involved as therapists, making the ordinary dialogue through which people learn about one another difficult. Despite the challenge, every clinician is faced with the job of making sense of patients' problems in order to form a plan to help, to develop a therapeutic relationship that allows adequate interventions, and to assess the progress and outcome of psychotherapy. Such a task requires a theory to organize what is observed—that is, a psychology of adolescence that can serve as an explanation of expected occurrences in the normal course of development and that may be used to understand deviations from the norm.

Some psychoanalytic theories are considered in this chapter in an attempt to provide an adequate framework for understanding a variety of specific complaints that relate to the adolescent's progress and problems in adaptation. A goal is to illustrate a broad and useful framework for understanding and treating adolescents that has resulted from the mutual influence of clinical experience, the considerable revisions of psychoanalytic theory, and research observation. Because the purpose is to present perspectives on the adolescent's psychological organization, the many social, cultural, and biological influences, including organic disorders, affecting learning, mood, and thought are not addressed directly, but are considered from the perspective of their meaning to the psychologically developing individual. The chapter is not intended to be an encyclopedic review of the considerable contributions to the psychoanalytic literature of adolescence. In addition, a single chapter could not possibly do justice to the rich and varied portraits of adolescence that have been drawn by psychotherapists, social scientists, artists, and writers. The interested reader is directed to such works as those by Greenspan and Pollock (1980) or Esman (1975, 1983) for a more in-depth exploration of the literature on adolescence.

Overview of Adolescence

Adolescence is the term that describes the period of human development between the end of the first and about the beginning of the third decades of life when a child transforms into a young person prepared for adulthood. It is generally accepted that adolescent development reflects the confluence of physical and cognitive maturation and the expectations of the adolescent, family, and society within an historical context. There are significant alterations in all aspects of life as the child explores new sexual and social behavior, new relationships with family and friends, and new intellectual skills.

Adolescence is usefully subdivided into three phases, during which time there may be a wide range and frequent shifting of moods and behavior (Miller 1983). Early in adolescence physical growth and sexual urges are a central preoccupation as the child experiences increased social and sexual opportunity and society's responses to the advent or the delayed arrival of secondary sexual characteristics. Privacy and extrafamilial contacts play an increasingly important role in the child's life. Relationships change in a fluctuating manner. At one moment friends and group affiliation play a central and valued role while parents are avoided and devalued, whereas at another moment the child may seek closeness to parents or seem to need them in childlike ways that have not been apparent for years. The child may feel vulnerable and experience moodiness and a fragile self-esteem.

Middle adolescence is a period of attention to a more specific definition of oneself. Ongoing social, sexual, and educational explorations are increasingly experienced within a context of self-definition. Independent thought and action are important in establishing oneself as unique and self determining. Emotions are intensely felt and often expressed with exquisite sensitivity as the adolescent increasingly forms a unique self perspective. Empathic appreciation of others in relationships is evident in caring, responsible behavior.

If all goes well, in late adolescence a self-sufficient, responsible young adult with a vastly changed self view and experience of others will ultimately emerge. The young adult will possess a realistic and resilient self concept that includes a reliable sense of values, ambitions, sexuality, and a balanced sense of uniqueness and affiliation with the surround. The new self concept will allow responsible reciprocal relationships with friends, family, and lovers and the ability to achieve satisfaction through expression in a number of activities.

The progressive changes in adolescent behavior are explained as the manifest expression of the developing child's efforts to master challenges and manage anxiety. Successful mastery is accomplished through the reorganization of typical patterns of experiencing oneself, others, and the world. The enduring patterns of psychological functions, or structures, that develop as a product of this reorganization are familiar as the shibboleths of adolescent development: identity, character, mature superego, and ego-ideal. Autonomy, individuation, and independence are attained as a most important concomitant of these structural changes.

There is general agreement that the transformations of adolescence are influenced by prior development, that reorganization presents the opportunity for new growth through recapitulation of earlier experience in light of new abilities, and that the transformations are molded by available avenues of expression. The progress toward mastery is monitored by reference to comfort with one's own body, the quality of relationships (with friends, family, and lovers), educational and, later, vocational vitality and direction, and the ability to plan flexibly and view responsibly one's life in the context of a generally positive and realistic attitude toward oneself and others. Because the achievement of self-maintenance and satisfying sexual, interpersonal, and vocational functioning are considered by adolescents and adults to be important to a productive and satisfying life, they are usually referred to as the *developmental tasks* of adolescence.

Theories of Adolescence

Explanations for the psychological transformations in adolescence have always been approached from within some general theoretical orientation of mental organization, development, and psychopathology. Each orientation has its own assumptions about the basic motivation for actions that organize psychological development and functioning. As a result, theories of drive, ego, separation-individuation, psychosocial interaction, or the development of the self make different contributions to the definition, the process, and the expected outcome of adolescence.

Adolescents were among Freud's first patients (Glenn 1980). Although not an adolescent psychiatrist, Freud's (1905/1953) focus on the psychosexual transformations of puberty formed the foundation for later elaborations of adolescent psychology. The most influential contributors to the psychosexual theory of adolescent development and psychopathology have rested their case on Freud's theory. Although there have been revisions of this theory to reflect the importance of conflict-free areas of development and of preoedipal adaptation, the preeminence of the sexual motive and conflict for development has remained.

In work most influential to understanding adolescent development, Blos (1962, 1979) classified the changes in instinct, ego, and superego into phases of adolescence that extend over roughly a 10-year span. The importance of instinctual discharge as the primary motivator for action is consonant with Blos's definition of adolescence as the change in psychological structures necessitated by puberty. In this view the primary task of adolescence is psychic restructuring necessitated by the sexual transformations of puberty. The transformation of instinct, ego, superego, and ego-ideal results in the formation of a stable character, an important aspect of which is affiliation with society. Adolescent behavior, then, is attributed to the regression and defenses arising out of restimulated oedipal conflict and withdrawal of libido from the threatening parental images back into the ego. Adolescence describes the process through which the child resolves these conflicts and develops a stable character structure within which personal definition and satisfying sexual discharge without overtaxing anxiety can proceed into adult life. The outcome of development depends on the child's ego strength, the strength of the instincts, and the adequacy of the child's defenses.

Adolescence begins as the result of a quantitative increase in instinctual pressure around puberty that is felt as a greater investment in all libidinal and aggressive modes of gratification. The child's ego is challenged as increasing instinctual pressure leads to a resurgence of earlier conflicts and modes of gratification previously repudiated by the superego. A regression ensues to early feelings of attachment and interest in the pregenital mother. For the boy, castration anxiety is restimulated and is often defended against by turning away from girls and intense investment in buddies and sports. The girl defends against the regressive pull to mother with a forceful turn toward heterosexuality.

In early adolescence as these processes continue, the child begins to withdraw interest in the parents as primary love objects, with a number of behavioral consequences related to the need to manage the now free-floating libidinal impulses. Withdrawal of libido from internalized parental images leaves the child with a sense of alienation. The guiding and stabilizing control of superego control by parental images is loosened, leaving the child subject to more erratic, irresponsible behavior. Increased narcissistic self preoccupation prior to investment in new, extra-familial sexual objects is responsible for the adolescent's grandiosity or low self-esteem as well as the over- or undervaluation of others. Parents are depreciated because their actual and internalized control over the child has been lessened. Furthermore, the identifications with the same-sex parent and repression of preoedipal bisexuality that marked the resolution of the oedipal phase in childhood are now no longer available. The adolescent develops intense erotic and idealizing relationships in an attempt to find objects for the impulses that are now free from investment in parental images. This search may be conceptualized as both shifting libidinal investment from one person to another, experienced as erotic desire, and the investment of self or narcissistic love in another, where the other is loved and emulated as an ideal. Homosexual fantasies and exploration may occur as the child shifts to a same-sex friend narcissistic libidinal investment that was previously attached to the preoedipal parent.

The idealization process in early adolescence is associated with the formation of the adult ego-ideal, a most important aspect of adolescent development. Idealizations are explained as the child's investment of narcissistic libido in others; that is, the self love that is increased as a result of the withdrawal of investment in others is now represented by viewing another as the self one wishes to be but cannot achieve. The qualities of the idealized object are exaggerated and the object is often felt to be unapproachable and intimidating. Whereas in childhood the oedipal phase was resolved with identification with the same-sex parent, repression of incestuous striving, and superego development, in adolescence a further transformation occurs in which the internalized parental standards represented in the superego are now revised. The more generalized controlling agency, the ego-ideal, allows greater autonomy and flexibility while continuing to give life meaning and regulate self-esteem.

With the beginning transformations of the ego-ideal and the engagement of object libido toward heterosexual object finding, adolescence proper begins. Two challenges mark this period and form the decisive tasks of adolescence: the final disengagement from primary love objects and the development of an adult identity (Blos 1962, 1967).

Masterson (1972), using object-relations theory, associated the adolescent's efforts to achieve autonomy with stable internal self and object representations, intact reality testing, and secure ego boundaries. He has described the adolescent's disengagement from primary love objects as a recapitulation of the separation-individuation phase of early childhood, allowed by the toddler's increased ability to differentiate self and object representations. During the separation-individuation phase the mother recognizes the infant's desire and ability to explore without her for periods of time as well as the child's periodic need to return for emotional refueling. As a result of this behavior the toddler assumes the ego functions originally supplied by the mother that ensure the child's autonomous functioning and positive self representations.

If the mother is unable to tolerate the child's press for autonomy but perceives the developmental thrust as an abandonment, she will withdraw emotional support, leaving the toddler feeling abandoned. The toddler, in turn, defends against the feelings of abandonment with ego splitting and denial and at the price of autonomy and its associated ego strengths. Later in life, around prepuberty, the child is again challenged with a normative thrust toward separation. Psychopathology is revealed at this point because the child is without the requisite internal structures to master the second individuation process.

Erikson (1968) emphasized identity as important to the integration of the person into the world of social interactions. Adolescence is a phase in an epigenetic view of identity formation when the child is faced with the challenge of functioning in a more complex world. Erikson views identity as a component term that is at once social and psychological. It refers to a "conscious sense of individual uniqueness . . . an unconscious striving for a continuity of experience . . . and a solidarity with a group's ideals" (p. 208). Erikson further explains that "one can then speak of ego identity when one discusses the ego's synthesizing power in the light of its central psychosocial function, and of self-identity when the integration of the individual's self- and role-images are under discussion" (p. 211).

Identity formation in adolescence represents a reworking and further application of childhood developmental achievements in light of current challenges and opportunities. Childhood issues of trust, self-maintenance and self-determination, imaginative play, and industrious activity are revisited as the adolescent forms an identity that includes the capacity for faith in and mutual recognition of others, group affiliation and role definition, a sense of one's unique qualities, and occupational choice. Furthermore, adolescent identity formation is associated with further development of intimacy, generativity, and integrity. Childhood failures to master the age-appropriate developmental tasks limit the adolescent's ability to commit to the challenges of physical maturation, occupational choice, and self-definition. The result is the psychopathology of identity confusion in adolescence. Identity confusion is marked by a number of symptoms. The adolescent fails to form intimate relationships and makes contacts that are self-enhancing, only to suffer disappointment and isolation at the inevitable disappointments. Concentration is poor and productive work is inhibited. The adolescent experiences an urgency for action and a lack of appreciation for time as a dimension of growth and change. A negative identity is formed that is defined by a rejection of all developmental expectations.

Anna Freud (1958) proposed that adolescence was by its nature a period of turmoil and that the absence of signs of regression and defense was itself an indication of psychopathology. She noted typical ego defenses that protect the adolescent from further regression and give this period its behavioral cast. The course of adolescence is normally stormy because strong sexual drives and an ego weakened by alienation from previous sources of superego equilibrium leave the child vulnerable to anxiety and regression. Anxiety caused by strong sensual impulses is associated with asceticism to renounce sensory experience completely. Intellectualization to render impulses under the control of words and logic or externalization to place fear and confusion beyond one's responsibility is frequently observed. In addition, Blos (1962) noted that uniformism—conforming to the dictates of a clique or philosophical stance—also serves to allow exploration of social or sexual behavior that might otherwise engender conflict and regression. This behavior may represent a defensive independence by virtue of oppositionality rather than a fluid exploration in the service of greater autonomy and self-definition. In such circumstances development is inhibited and the adolescent's behavior is shallow and unfulfilling.

Character consolidation, the end result of the adolescent process, is increasingly evident in late adolescence and marks the final resolution of conflict and defense (Blos 1968). As the adolescent works toward mastering restimulated conflicts and achieves increased autonomy, intense affects become more modulated and fluctuating behaviors more consistent. The adolescent is more realistic and is now introspective in a way that demonstrates a greater appreciation and acceptance of one's strengths and limitations. A more clearly defined person emerges as the unique mixture of conflict and modes of resolution and defense are elaborated, stabilized, and integrated into a pattern of overall functioning.

The final cast of character consolidation is the result of the synthesis of all the factors previously described. Early trauma that has been reworked may leave its mark as sensitivities that are now ego syntonic, integrated into rather than threatening overall adaptive functioning. The degree to which separation from infantile object ties has been mastered is reflected in assured self assertion and comfortable choices involving work, intimate relationships, and personal values. Clear sexual identity enables one to pursue sexual partners without undue ambivalence or anxiety over the normal regression during sexual behavior. The late adolescent's ability to achieve maximal integration and perspective allows a sense of oneself as continuous and whole over time despite variations and further change in life's experiences. Failure to achieve character consolidation may result from failure of the ego's integrative capacities and flexibility, overwhelming pressures of impulses, or extreme demands from the environment (Blos 1968).

Finally, the end of adolescence is marked by a further integration and acceptance of one's self as unique yet with a comfortable place in the world. Residual conflicts and sensitivities continue to be worked on in the context of consistent self-definition, giving life a particular emphasis, but without threatening disruptive loss of functioning.

Adolescence has also been approached by self psychology as a period of self reorganization involving transformations of ideals and ambitions. The theory of self psychology is organized around the importance of empathic persons who are capable of fostering the needed selfobject experiences necessary to form the basis of a cohesive self (Kohut 1971, 1977, 1984). Kohut's early clinical descriptions relied on ego psychology to postulate separate lines of libido and narcissism. He later abandoned instinct theory and developed a theory with the self as the main organizer of behavior and motivation and empathic selfobjects as central to development. Satisfying sexual expression and indeed self assertions in relationships and tasks of all kinds reflect stable selfobject experiences.

Kohut's theory is that infants grow in the context of caregivers who are more or less empathic, enabling or thwarting the realization of ambitions and ideals in combination with talents. Early in life the child develops a grandiose self that requires mirroring from caregivers and an idealizing self that forms idealizations of caregivers as perfect beings. Failure of the caregivers to provide adequate empathic relations to the child results in a fragility of the child's grandiose or idealizing self and a failure of his or her modification and transformation into mature selfobject relatedness with a healthy self-esteem. As a result, the child may disavow or split off one aspect of his or her self. Over time this disavowed self continues to seek satisfying selfobject experiences, coloring future adult relationships. The person cannot appreciate others as having an independent center of initiative, but continues to view others as extensions of one's self where the purpose is to provide the missing selfobject experience. Treatment in this model involves repairing the split in the person's psyche so that he or she becomes aware of the archaic grandiosity or idealizations and can, in a more empathic environment of optimal disillusionment, internalize a more realistic view of self and others and attain more mature selfobject experiences.

Kohut's theory that the development of a cohesive self is based on the internalization of idealized and mirroring parental images led him to propose the central role of the transformation of ideals in the reorganization of the self during adolescence (Kohut 1972). Following Kohut's lead, Wolf et al. (1972) reviewed the essential characteristics of the adolescent process and proposed an outline of the transformations during adolescence. They proposed that adolescence is not a reaction to puberty, but rather that "the essential requirement for its occurrence seems to be the emergence of an inner necessity for new ideals, accompanied by opportunities encountered for such a transformation of the self" (p. 269).

The need for new ideals is precipitated by young persons' increasing ability to view their parents and themselves more realistically, making the standards and values developed in childhood less useful, by increasing cognitive maturation and by increasing opportunities and demands of society. The transformation to new ideals follows a predictable sequence initiated by a phase appropriate de-idealization of parental standards. The loss of these internalized standards is experienced as turmoil and is managed through the formation of intense peer relations in the service of maintaining narcissistic equilibrium. Peer groups may serve mirroring or idealizing selfobject functions and allow the safe expression of grandiosity and exploration of new ideals. The particular form of the selfobject need may relate to efforts to overcome prior disappointments in childhood selfobject experiences. As adolescents form unique new ideals and avenues for their expression, the need for the selfobject functions of peers diminishes and relationships are discarded or become more ordinary.

Wolf (1982) emphasized the point that these relationships are not simply opportunities to explore new social roles but that they provide important stabilizing parts to a changing psychic structure. The need for selfobject experiences continues throughout life, although the intensity of the need for self stabilization may vary depending on life's circumstances.

Marohn (1977) notes that in delinquent adolescents the normal process of de-idealization, experimentation with one's own grandiosity, and affiliation with peers as sources of mirroring and idealizing selfobject experiences is precluded. The low self-esteem, lack of ambition, callous use of others, brutal grandiosity, severe disillusionment, rage, and fragmentation with frantic activity in delinquent patients may be understood as narcissistic pathology. It is not the emergence of sexual and aggressive feelings but the accompanying shifts in grandiosity and idealizations that threaten the adolescent. The restimulated archaic selfobject needs associated with these shifts create the anxiety associated with the fear of self fragmentation. The emergence of grandiosity and idealizations may serve as both defenses against low self-esteem and desperate efforts to cling to much needed archaic idealizing and mirroring selfobject ties.

Sklansky (1977) employed Kohut's separation of libidinal and narcissistic developmental lines and the concept of idealization and mirroring to clarify the evolving nature of love relationships in adolescence. The intensity of adolescent love relationships suggests their importance in maintaining narcissistic equilibrium during the transformations of the period. In early adolescence idealizations predominate as the adolescent seeks stabilizing selfobject experiences while parents are devalued and revived oedipal longings remain repressed. The predominance of idealizations in early adolescence may help clarify homosexual behavior common during this period. It is not the sex of the person but his or her ability to provide stability and vitality to the self that is important. Later, erotic pleasure is more central, but orgasm remains important not only for release of sexual tension but also for self confirmation. Mature love is a developmental achievement that involves zonal pleasures and affirmation of the wholeness of self experience.

Influences of Revisions in Psychoanalytic Theory on Approaches to Adolescence

As mentioned, adolescence has been understood in the context of a general theory of motivation and development. There are a number of such models, each with its own assumptions about the basic motivation for actions that organize psychological development and functioning (Greenberg and Mitchell 1983). In turn, these assumptions result in different emphases on the definition, the process of psychological transformations, and the expected outcome of adolescence.

For example, psychoanalytic theories that follow Freud's emphasis on the biphasic nature of sexual development with instinctual discharge as the primary motivator for action view adolescence primarily as the necessary revision of childhood sexuality in response to puberty. Independence, identity, intimacy, and realistic productivity reflect the successful transformation of oedipal and preoedipal conflict so that the mature expression of sexual impulses is assured. Other psychoanalytic theories that emphasize the primacy of object relatedness and self and object differentiation for motivation view adolescence as the manifestation of efforts to achieve self sufficiency, or autonomy, with stable internal objects. Yet another theory is organized around the importance of empathic relations with others that form the basis of a stable self. In this view, adolescence is a period of self reorganization involving transformations of ideals and ambitions resulting in mature relatedness. Satisfying self assertions in relationships and in tasks of all kinds reflect stable selfobject experiences.

Each theory emphasizes some aspect of adolescence, and together they provide a sense of the rich tapestry of the adolescent process. Problems arise, however, when one looks more carefully at the individual theories or attempts to integrate them. To many practitioners, the theory of adolescence may often seem as impenetrable as the adolescents it purports to explain, fluctuating as it does between a focus on childhood and adulthood, between psychic structure and fitting into the social surround, and between sexual and aggressive drives and the importance of ideals. To add to the problem the data of observation, the behavior of adolescents, continue to be elaborated. The complexities and limitations of theory and technique have left many therapists with an uneasy relationship to the theory that explains patients' behavior. They may feel restricted if they force their understanding into a framework that seems inadequate to describe and treat the problems they encounter, or alienated as they work pragmatically and flexibly but with a sense of operating outside or or in opposition to standard practice.

For a number of years extensive attention has been devoted to clarifying the psychoanalytic theory of motivation and development and to providing a useful theory of therapy. Changes in psychoanalytic thinking have involved the reciprocal influence of investigations of motivation, theory formation, new discoveries in clinical process and technique, and observational research. These findings have been usefully applied to a broader understanding of adolescence.

Freud's method of theory formation has been vigorously criticized, and his basic assumptions about thought and motivation have been examined and revised.[1] Freud's assumption was that mental functioning consists of sexual and aggressive instincts driving a closed-system mental apparatus with the aim of tension discharge regulated by the pleasure principle (Basch 1988). In his theory the infant is a bundle of needs and reflexes who must begin to relate to other people in order to survive because wish fulfillment is inadequate to sustain life. Developmental stages culminating in the capacity for love, work, and play are the result of com-

---

[1]Although it is beyond the scope of this chapter to include a discussion of the many cogent criticisms of Freud's metapsychology and theory formation, the interested reader is directed to the scholarly work of Basch (1973, 1977) for discussions of theory formation and explanatory theory, and G. Klein (1976) for an examination of clinical theory and metapsychology. Also, Schafer (1976, 1983) has examined the issues of identity, character, and self in light of modifications in Freudian metapsychology.

plex transformations of instinct under the influence of the controlling agencies of ego, superego, and ego-ideal.

Freud thought of libido as an energy pressing for discharge, originally invested in oneself as narcissistic libido. Later, libido is invested in objects in the service of obtaining gratification not possible if one's self is the only object. There is a natural progression of oral, anal, phallic, and genital modes of libidinal investment in objects. Such basic issues as the development of reality testing, the formation of intimate relationships, and the use of guiding ideals and values are seen as methods of ensuring discharge of libidinal energy without undue anxiety or conflict.

In contrast to Freud's views, child observation studies have demonstrated that infants enter the world as information processing and organizing individuals who are very responsive to the environment (Lichtenberg 1982, 1983; Stern 1985). Affective communication and the search for order serve as a more useful concept for motivation than does instinct (Basch 1976). Development is more usefully understood to proceed from the fact that the brain integrates information rather than seen as a need to ensure instinctual discharge and to avoid danger. Information ordinarily is included or excluded from awareness depending on its importance to the person's ongoing competent functioning, and important information may be excluded if it threatens functioning (Basch 1983).

In addition to the motivational theory of instinct, Freud assumed that infants' thinking included symbols in much the same way that adults use words. Thinking was not responsive to reality, however, but was governed by primary process. Only later, under the influence of the reality principle did secondary process, or logical thought, occur. Piaget (Piaget and Inhelder 1969) demonstrated that infants do not think like adults, but go through a progression of cognitive changes involving the increasingly complex use and manipulation of symbols. That these modes of thought are not like adults makes them no less reality oriented. These revisions of the basic assumptions about human thought and motivation significantly affect any theory of development, defenses, and psychopathology.

The theory of adolescence has also been influenced by discoveries from the clinical process. Observations of transference, countertransference, and necessary alterations in technique have broadened our understanding of factors that affect therapeutic change. For example, clinical intervention in classical psychoanalysis was aimed primarily at the interpretation of unconscious oedipal or preoedipal conflict. Many patients, however, could not comply with the usual process of reporting thoughts, feelings, dreams, and associations. Transference issues seemed directed to the patient-therapist relationship and could not be profitably managed by interpretation of defense, resistance, or conflict. Many patients needed special accommodations in order to tolerate the therapeutic process (Eissler 1953). For these patients, progress in treatment seemed more connected to the stabilizing effects of the relationship than to insight into repressed wishes. From a theoretical standpoint, the importance of the patient-therapist relationship in therapeutic change encouraged clinicians to look for an explanation for these phenomena in that period of life involving the emergence of a self-sufficient individual. From a clinical standpoint clinicians were encouraged to view these phenomena as transferences in their own right and not simply as resistance.

Kohut (1971) shifted the emphasis in psychoanalysis from a mechanistic and resistance-oriented view of patients' behavior to viewing transferences as attempts to complete a process of achieving a sense of wholeness. Kohut's work began as a reaction against the mechanical style of analysts who used ego psychology and viewed all phenomena as related to psychosexual conflict and all patients' problems in treatment as resistance to bringing unconscious material into the transference. Kohut observed that some of his patients did not seem troubled by psychosexual conflict, but seemed to be trying to realize other unmet childhood needs. He termed these manifestations in his patients *mirroring* and *idealizing* transferences. He found that if he did not interpret these attitudes of his patients toward him as evasions of oedipal conflict, but allowed patients to use him in these ways, they improved considerably.

Clinicians have always been aware that adolescents are difficult to engage and that they work poorly in an environment that demands careful attention to introspection, verbal modes of expression, and a fairly high degree of self-control. They have also long been aware that adolescents often change as a result of allying with admired adults who supply a consistent environment rather than insight (Aichhorn 1925; Marohn 1977). Kohut's contributions have been especially useful in understanding adolescent grandiosity and idealizations and the special therapeutic challenges particular to the transformations of adolescence (Wolf 1980). In addition, the shift in focus to the subjective experience of the individual striving for wholeness has been especially salutary for understanding the adolescent's need for guidance, genuine affective responses, help in forming a realistic assessment of themselves and others, and the need for a range of interventions with adolescent patients (Goldberg 1978).

In addition to an increased understanding of adolescents derived from the clinical setting, behavioral observations in nonclinical populations have significantly influenced the theory of the adolescent process. Psychoanalytic theory developed to explain psychopathology and was then extended to include a general theory of mental life. In recent years extensive research focusing on social (Csikszentmihalyi and Larson 1984), cultural (Havinghurst 1987), and political (Gallatin 1980) behaviors during adolescence has called into question some important observations on which the theory of adolescence has rested. Offer and Offer's (1975) longitudinal study of adolescent development is an example.

Offer questioned the transposition of a theory derived from troubled adolescents to a theory of normal adolescent development. Psychoanalytic theory suggested that because the oedipal conflict was restimulated during puberty, the erratic, alienated, action-oriented, and self-absorbed behavior of adolescents was normal and that behavior that would be interpreted as abnormal in any other period was seen in adolescence as normal and even desirable (A. Freud 1958). As a result, diagnosis of pathology in adolescence was quite difficult. Offer's work delineated three general routes through adolescence that he termed *continuous, surgent,* and *tumultuous,* clarifying that not all adolescents experience turmoil and that the absence of turmoil does not indicate developmental pathology. Masterson (1967) also demonstrated that although many adolescents experience some disruption in relationships and fluctuations in behavior, psychopathology is as clearly distinguishable in adolescence as in other phases of life.

These observations have been useful clinically in cautioning therapists not to dismiss adolescent misbehavior or symptoms as part of a normative crisis. In addition, the finding that intense sensual experience during adolescence is not necessarily associated with significant disruptions in the continuity of adolescent relationships or overall functioning has emphasized the importance of self regulation and continuity rather than sexual impulses and oedipal conflict in a theory of adolescent psychopathology.

A Revised Conceptualization of the Adolescent Process

Basch (1988) incorporated the theoretical, clinical, and research advances in psychoanalytic thinking in developing a theory to organize clinical observations that may be usefully applied to understanding adolescent development and psychopathology. It is of further use in providing a rationale for the wide spectrum of interventions employed with adolescents. The reader may not be as familiar with this model as with more classical formulations that treat adolescence as a recapitulation of oedipal and preoedipal conflict with regression stimulated by sexual impulses. In order to provide the context for understanding the changes of adolescence within this system, a brief summary of this developmental model is presented below.

In this view development may be understood as the achievement of competent functioning through the integration of increasingly complex information (particularly information experienced through the affects) allowed by cognitive maturation within the context of an empathic environment. The basis for the developmental theory is that motivation is based on the brain's function of organizing information in the service of adaptation, a process Basch (1988) refers to as the *self system*:

> Life on any level—vegetative, psychological, or social—depends on the ability of the organism to adapt to the environment that makes possible existence, or some aspect of it. This adaptation necessitates the continuous process of signals by interrelated, error-correcting feedback cycles. Together these feedback cycles form hierarchical organizations of systems that monitor the environment and adjust themselves to it. (p. 104)

Basch goes on to add:

> Self system is a collective term encompassing the hierarchy of neurologically encoded, goal-directed feedback cycles whose activity constitutes character and governs behavior. (p. 106)

From birth there is an error-correcting feedback cycle between caregivers and infants whereby the infant learns. Information from internal and environmental sources is received, amplified, and communicated through an inborn system of affects that include startle, interest, anger, pleasure, distress, disgust, and fear. Although the mode of learning changes through development, progressing from preverbal sensorimotor modes of cognition to abstract thought, the affective tone of that which is learned determines the meaning it will have for the child. It is this affective meaning that becomes part of the self system and that will influence later motivation for actions.

These very early interactions that combine learning in a particular affective tone become the patterns of expectation with which new information is met and that determine how new information will be understood and what response will occur. (For most interesting elaborations of self development in infancy see Lichtenberg [1983, 1989] and Stern [1985].) Whenever the child is met with something new he or she attempts to make a match with something already known in order to feel a continuous sense of integration and be able to muster an effective response. If there is a match it is experienced as competence. When there is a mismatch the infant will continue to try responses until a match can be made, but may eventually become agitated or apathetic. If all goes well, the infant is able to develop within a context in which he or she feels effective in eliciting predictable responses that can be integrated as self experiences.

When the child reaches about 18 months these patterns of experience with their associated emotional tone become symbolized in words as feelings, and the child can evoke them in the absence of an immediate stimulus. The child may now be said to have a concept of self, or the ability to transform overall goal-oriented experience, self-system functioning, into a symbolic representation. Once the self concept is in place, the child can use it to assess information in terms of its relevance to the self system in order to ensure competent functioning. The conscious feeling of pleasure associated with effective self functioning is termed self-esteem.

There is increasing differentiation between child and caregivers as the child becomes competent with independent care during this period. The child develops an increasing ability to coordinate goals and operate in an overall integrated fashion. However, the child's ability to experience competence through maintaining himself or herself will remain dependent on the responses of caregivers for some time. To maintain an integrated self concept and a self system that remains open to new information, the child utilizes the affectively attuned responses of supportive and encouraging caregivers. The child's internal experiences of these relationships that help to maintain the integrity of self functioning are termed mirroring and idealizing selfobject experiences.

Over the next few years the child is increasingly able to maintain himself or herself in an overall integrated fashion without parental assistance. Whereas in the previous period preoperational thought allowed the child to maintain integration by ignoring the affective significance of incompatible information or aims through disavowal and to maintain an idealized view of caregivers, the child now has a more realistic understanding of caregivers and protects himself or herself by excluding affectively significant information from conscious awareness (Basch 1977). With the advent of concrete operations in cognitive functioning the child can use repression to reconcile conflicting interests and preserve self competence. The child makes increasing use of learned standards of behavior rather than the approval of an idealized or mirroring parental image for approval. The accepted set of standards allows the child greater latitude for action outside the immediate vicinity of the parents while maintaining self competence.

A variety of circumstances may be associated with problems in affective attunement necessary for the child to make adequate use of selfobject experiences. In an erratic environment or in one absent of stimulation the infant cannot develop clear patterns of expectation and response that lead to competence and self stability. There may also be problems when the infant lacks the ability to process ordinary communications as a result of some neurological deficit or from differences in temperament between parents and the infant.

Perhaps more common is a problem that arises when aspects of the infant-caregiver interaction are so unique that they are not usable in a more general context. A moment that offers the potential for greater integration becomes instead a threat to the relationship with the caregiver and reinforces a continued need for the child to remain within the context of the original situation in order to feel competent. In such circumstances, at a moment of self assertion about a state or a need, the child is forced to ignore what is naturally felt and substitute a different person's response. The child, rather than having had new information and explorations be met with affirmation, may have found it impossible to integrate new experiences either because the skills for managing the new experience had not been taught or because to engage the new experience would have threatened a needed mode of organizing one's self (Gedo 1988).

In the future when similar circumstances arise they are experienced as disruptive because they are humiliating or threaten the loss of integration once again. When that happens the person may use a variety of means to exclude new information that might restimulate the anxiety of a failing self system. Depending on the child's resources and the developmental period of the original disruption, these means may be withdrawal or more complex behaviors such as projective identification, disavowal, or repression. The particular defense employed to protect the child's functioning probably relates to the child's cognitive abilities and the degree to which the child had a solidly integrated self cohesion during the period when problematic experiences were encountered.

Gedo (1979, 1988) has organized a number of clinical phenomena into an epigenetic theory of self-organization that relates to states of behavioral function and dysfunction. When the period of problems relates to the earliest development of a self fluctuating in the ability to maintain a coherent set of goals, issues of splitting, projective identification, separation, and abandonment may apply. If the problems occur later, when the child is better able to maintain overall integration and competence but is still in need of caregiver support to maintain integrated functioning, narcissistic vulnerability and relationships marked by disavowal, grandiosity, or idealizations may dominate the clinical picture. Still later, usually when the child has also progressed to be able to think using more complex manipulations of symbols and when issues of sexuality and competition emerge in a more reliably intact self, repression of unacceptable impulses may be the prominent defense. Another way to describe these stages is to say that development involves learning to regulate tension, develop a coherent plan of self-monitored activity, come to grips with reality over illusion, and channel desires appropriately (Gedo 1988). Foreclosure of any of these adaptive achievements may result in psychopathology.

This developmental approach may be extended into adolescence. Within a model that views development as the progressive integration of increasingly complex information allowed by cognitive maturation within the context of an empathic environment, adolescence is a period of necessary change to accommodate greater complexity. Between the second and third decades of life the young person is challenged to integrate a number of occurrences within the self system. Lichtenberg (1982) notes a number of activities that maintain continuity with early development but are significantly altered during adolescence. These include biophysiological regulation (eating, sleeping, eliminating), perceptual-cognitive developments (play and work), interactive behavior (socializing), regulation of bodily tension coordinated with gender identity (sexuality), and affectively charged behavior patterns (thrills and risks). The need to develop new skills in adolescence with respect to bodily functions, interpersonal relationships, and ideals and values requires expanding the range of the cohesive self. Lichtenburg notes that since the establishment of a cohesive self and the capacity for symbolic logic (cognitive maturation) are childhood tasks that do not need to be remastered in adolescence, they provide the adolescent with abilities not available in early life through which continuing issues may be reworked. Problems from childhood in these areas may therefore be advantageously revised during the adolescent process.

The adolescent process may be considered in terms of the shifting equilibrium of the self system—that is, in terms of the developing child's ability to remain open to new affect-laden information. The emphasis on adolescence as a major reorganization of the self system in the service of maintaining competence helps organize the various definitions of adolescence as biological, psychological, cognitive, and social phenomena within a subjective perspective rather than one of external observation. Thus, adolescence is not defined by any of the component phenomena of the period, but rather by the meaning of the changes to the young person (Gedo 1979). Such a conceptualization of adolescence that separates the physical from the psychological transformations during the second decade of life is consistent with the clinical finding that some postpubertal people remain psychologically frozen in latency (Gedo 1979) and with the historical perspective that adolescence as it is currently experienced is a recent historical phenomenon (Rakoff 1989).

Tension regulation, organizing one's self according to a coherent plan, placing reality over illusion, and exploring appropriate avenues to channel desires are particularly related to mastery of the tasks of adolescence. If the necessary revisions in any of these areas are blocked because new challenges threaten to disrupt a cohesive self, problems in adaptation may ensue. A number of symptoms and phenomena of the adolescent period have been reexamined in light of the idea that failures to adapt to new affect-laden information represent the inability to match the information with preexisting expectations and thus result in increased anxiety and confusion.

For example, Gedo (1979) notes that intellectualization, obsessional preoccupation, hypochondriasis, and asceticism may be understood as the manifestations of attempts to preserve a failing self-organization. The particular symptom reflects the degree to which the self is disorganized and the self concept is concretized as physical. General symptoms such as lethargy, emptiness, or periods of hopelessness may be the manifestations of fluctuating self-organization. Obsessional concerns represent a heightened self awareness. The adolescent may obsess about alternatives (doubting) but still has a self concept as one who is still able to select between various alternatives. Or, the very ability to be a problem solver may come into question with a preoccupation with the mechanics of mental functions. Hypochondriasis represents a self experience as actual body functioning with loss of the symbolizing capacity and a return to operating in a sensorimotor mode.

Influences of Developmental Theory on the Theory of Psychotherapy

One of the important outcomes of the revisions of the theory of motivation and development has been to make motivational and developmental theory more consistent with a theory of psychotherapy that encompasses a variety of flexibly employed techniques. It has already been stated that development involves the progressive integration of increasingly complex information from internal and external sources allowed by cognitive maturation within the context of an empathic environment. The integration of information occurs through an error-correcting feedback cycle of information processing, or self system, present from birth (Basch 1988). The ability to continue to integrate new experiences throughout life depends on the establishment of a cohesive self that can process new information in light of its affective significance without threat to competence, an ability subjectively experienced as self-esteem. Self cohesion may be understood as a progressive developmental achievement spanning the second year to about the sixth year of life and as part of a sequence of self-reorganization (Gedo 1979). Self cohesion is enabled by a variety of experiences, especially affirming and encouraging relationships with caregivers who are affectively attuned to the child's developmental needs and abilities (Kohut 1984). Mirroring or idealizing validation of the self refers to the child's internal experience of relationships that serve to ensure overall integrated functioning. Once reliable self cohesion is established, relationships that provide stabilizing selfobject experiences become less necessary under ordinary circumstances. However, during various occurrences throughout life, such as traumatic events or expectable transitions such as adolescence, relationships that provide selfobject functions may again become paramount. The ability to effectively make use of relationships to provide stable selfobject functions during these periods depends on the outcome of previous similar efforts.

Basch (1988) has aptly described psychotherapy as applied developmental psychology. Consistent with this view, psychotherapy seeks to help remove the obstacles to competent functioning through empathic immersion in the patient's subjective experience and an explanation of the patient's efforts to adapt. The fulcrum for change is the establishment of a relationship wherein the patient is able to use the therapist to enable self stability, to recruit appropriate selfobject experiences, during the therapeutic process.

Psychotherapy with adolescents is usefully viewed within the framework of psychotherapy as applied developmental psychology. The young person's need and desire to meet the tasks of adolescence results in a period of self-disorganization that necessitates the use of stabilizing experiences. The adolescent's ability to maintain self functioning and to use selfobjects during the time of transition determines how this period of transformation is negotiated. Teachers, friends, rock stars, literary figures, and a variety of other relationships and activities may be used to serve a mirroring or idealizing function, eroticized or not, in the service of maintaining and revising self functioning. In psychotherapy the new selfobject experience may itself be therapeutic (Kohut 1984) or may serve as an important part of the environment that provides the context for learning new skills (Gedo 1988). This is the case when adolescents present with learning, mood, or physical disorders. The stabilizing selfobject experiences enable the adolescent to maintain self functioning and self-esteem while learning new skills consistent with his or her abilities.

Resistance and regression in psychotherapy are viewed as manifestations of the patient's inability to make productive selfobject use of the therapist because experiences in the therapy revive previous traumatic or failed selfobject experiences that once again threaten self cohesion. Gedo's (1979) enumeration of a number of symptoms and behaviors that others have commonly attributed to adolescents serves as a relevant example of symptoms classified by progressive self-disorganization. Some adolescents may manifest the earliest sensorimotor patterns in addictions or they may become hypochondriacal or obsessional. Other adolescents with more resilient self cohesion may experience revived incestuous wishes primarily and may use action in the service of keeping these from consciousness. Consistent with Offer's continuous growth group, some adolescents may even be able to continue to make use of their own parents during the transformation. Failure to find any avenue for self-maintenance may result in major depression or suicide (Basch 1975).

The approach to psychotherapeutic intervention that follows from this model is one that enables the adolescent to experience competence by helping the patient to articulate, organize, and integrate an increasingly complex life. In psychotherapy, patients form images of their therapists as threatening objects of suspicion, devalued parents, admired teachers, allies against society, worthy partners to debate philosophical issues, or erotic and idealized sexual partners. These are not merely transferences that represent defenses against repressed libidinal wishes. They are the patient's attempts to use the therapist to develop self experiences that help reestablish and maintain a failing sense of organization and direction.

The shift in emphasis from conflict to efforts at overall self development and competent functioning includes empathic understanding of the patient's subjective experiences (Goldberg 1978). Empathic understanding is the process through which one comes to appreciate the affective as well as cognitive experiences of another (Basch 1983). Through the therapist's synthesis of affective resonance with the patient's communications, interpretation of the resonance in light of the therapist's own experiences, and the evaluation of the personal meaning of the communication within the larger context of the therapist's knowledge of the patient, the experiential state of the patient may be ascertained.

The issue of empathic understanding with adolescents in psychotherapy is significant in two ways. First, it may be difficult to feel emotionally in tune with adolescents in psychotherapy. Their action orientation, self preoccupation, reluctance or inability to engage in a dialogue where expression and mutual understanding of personal meaning is a goal, and fluctuating emotional integration all make resonance difficult. It can be helpful to know that the process of empathic understanding can begin with any of the components of resonance, interpretation, or evaluation. For example, it is often necessary to begin an understanding of adolescents through a thought experiment in which the therapist wonders how he or she would feel in the patient's circumstances. Similarly, the therapist may begin the process of mutual understanding by talking about his or her general knowledge of what kind of struggles young people typically encounter in growing up, knowledge the therapist has derived from studies of adolescent development and psychopathology. Second, adolescence itself is a time of maturation of the empathic appreciation of other's emotions. Basch (1983) describes a developmental sequence of affect (an autonomically mediated communication system), feeling (the word-labeling of affect), emotion (the combination of feelings), and empathy, that reaches maturation in adolescence. Empathic understanding involves the ability to decenter, or objectively view one's own emotions and appreciate another's. It is enhanced by the advent of formal operations (Piaget and Inhelder 1969). Not only, then, is empathic understanding the route to appreciating the adolescent patient's subjective world, but it is also something the adolescent is learning and for which the therapist's behavior and the very process of therapy serve as a model.

Therapists have creatively employed a variety of interventions to help adolescents regain competent functioning. Until late adolescence, development typically occurs more through exploration than reflection, so that often a therapist is required to be quite active. The therapist may be used to give direct advice, provide information about sex, discuss educational or vocational opportunities, act as a sounding board for exploring the possibility and planning of new ideas and actions, make self disclosure about his or her own feelings, offer a consistent and dependable set of values, or help develop a realistic acceptance of strengths and limitations. Interpretation of unconscious conflict expressed through action or in symbolic form also plays a role but, unlike many treatments with adults, is not usually primary.

Descriptions of psychotherapeutic aims and techniques with adolescents based on the classical psychoanalytic model have emphasized synthesis over analysis (Gitelson 1948) or the provision of ego support over the expression of regressive wishes and conflict (Meeks 1971; Masterson 1958). Although flexibility and availability are recommended, an integrated rationale for the full range of interventions has been lacking. Gedo and Goldberg (1973) offer a useful schema that organizes interventions according to the developmental level of the patient's self-organization. There are three types of interventions in addition to interpretation. *Pacification* is the provision of a soothing and consistent environment and may be indicated when an adolescent is functioning without the capacity for verbal expression or self-reflection. This is often the case with severely disturbed or psychotic adolescents who are unable to control their behavior or communicate through enactments. *Unification* involves presenting oneself as a real and affectively responsive person to help the adolescent reestablish an organized and coordinated plan of activity when self cohesion is disrupted. *Optimal frustration* may be used when the adolescent is functioning with a fairly stable self cohesion but needs help with functioning realistically without self-sustaining illusions.

Of particular value was Gedo and Goldberg's observation that in any treatment, any patient, no matter how well integrated, shifts between modes of integration and requires all of these types of interventions. What distinguishes a patient diagnostically is the most evident or typical mode of organization. Such a flexible stance is well suited for adolescence, when fluctuations between infantile and adult modes of behavior and self concept are frequent and the therapist is required to maintain empathic contact with patients by understanding and intervening according to these sometimes momentary shifts.

Conclusions

Adolescence is a period of transformation from childhood and preparation for adulthood. It involves changes in every area of a young person's emotional and interactional life. There have been a number of theoretical orientations that have been applied to understanding adolescent development and to developing a theory of psychotherapy.

In order for a theory to be valuable to the clinician it must provide an understanding of normal development in which a variety of specific complaints and problems in adaptation may be understood. In addition, it should provide a consistent integration of theories of motivation, development, and treatment. This chapter has served as an overview of psychoanalytic adolescent psychology and of revisions that have influenced our understanding of the adolescent process of transformation. A model that integrates revisions of theory, advances in clinical practice, and the yield of observational research is offered that may be applied to understanding adolescence and to a theory of psychotherapy that affords a variety of interventions flexibly employed. It is not possible to provide any final statement of adolescent behavior or theory. Like the adolescent struggling with the reality of the probabilistic nature of life, the reader must be prepared to struggle with the fact that we are still describing adolescence and developing a theory that will adequately capture the complex tapestry of human development, of which the adolescent experience is only a part.

References

Aichhorn A: Wayward Youth. New York, Viking Press, 1925

Basch MF: Psychoanalysis and theory formation. Annual of Psychoanalysis 1:9–52, 1973

Basch MF: Towards a theory that encompasses depression: a revision of existing causal hypothesis in psychoanalysis, in Depression and Human Existence. Edited by Anthony J, Benedek T. Boston, MA, Little, Brown, 1975, pp 483–534

Basch MF: The concept of affect: a re-examination. J Am Psychoanal Assoc 24:759–777, 1976

Basch MF: Developmental psychology and explanatory theory in psychoanalysis. Annual of Psychoanalysis 5:229–263, 1977

Basch MF: Empathic understanding: a review of the concept and some theoretical considerations. J Am Psychoanal Assoc 31:101–126, 1983

Basch MF: Understanding Psychotherapy. New York, Basic Books, 1988

Blos P: On Adolescence. Glencoe, IL, Free Press, 1962

Blos P: The second individuation process of adolescence. Psychoanal Study Child 22:162–186, 1967

Blos P: Character formation in adolescence. Psychoanal Study Child 23:245–263, 1968

Blos P: Modifications in the classical psychoanalytic model of adolescence. Adolesc Psychiatry 7:6–25, 1979

Csikszentmihalyi M, Larson R: Being Adolescent. New York, Basic Books, 1984

Eissler K: The effect of the structure of the ego on psychoanalytic technique. J Am Psychoanal Assoc 1:104–143, 1953

Erikson E: Identity: Youth and Crisis. New York, WW Norton, 1968

Esman A (ed): The Psychology of Adolescence: Essential Readings. New York, International Universities Press, 1975

Esman A (ed): The Psychiatric Treatment of Adolescents. New York, International Universities Press, 1983

Freud A: Adolescence. Psychoanal Study Child 13:255–278, 1958

Freud S: Three essays on the theory of sexuality (1905), in The Standard Edition of the Complete Psychological Works of Sigmund Freud, Vol 7. Translated and edited by Strachey J. London, Hogarth Press, 1953, pp 123–245

Gallatin J: Political thinking in adolescence, in Handbook of Adolescent Psychology. Edited by Adelson J. New York, John Wiley, 1980, pp 344–382

Gedo J: Beyond Interpretation. New York, International Universities Press, 1979

Gedo J: The Mind in Disorder. New York, Analytic Press, 1988

Gedo J, Goldberg A: Models of the Mind. Chicago, IL, University of Chicago Press, 1973

Gitelson M: Character synthesis: the psychotherapeutic problem of adolescence. Am J Orthopsychiatry 18:422–431, 1948

Glenn J; Freud's adolescent patients: Katharina Dora and the "homosexual woman," in Freud and His Patients. Edited by Kanzer M, Glenn J. New York, Jason Aronson, 1980, pp 23–47

Goldberg A: A shift in emphasis: adolescent psychotherapy and the psychology of the self. Journal of Youth and Adolescence 7:119–134, 1978

Greenberg J, Mitchell S: Object Relations in Psychoanalytic Theory. Cambridge, MA, Harvard University Press, 1983

Greenspan S, Pollock G (eds): The Course of Life: Psychoanalytic Contributions Towards Understanding Personality Development, Vol 2: Latency, Adolescence and Youth, Adelphi, MD, U.S. Department of Health and Human Services, 1980

Havinghurst R: Adolescent culture and subculture, in Handbook of Adolescent Psychology. Edited by Von Hasselt VB, Hersen M. New York, Pergamon Press, 1987, pp 401–412

Klein GS: Psychoanalytic Theory. New York, International Universities Press, 1976

Kohut H: The Analysis of the Self. New York, International Universities Press, 1971

Kohut H: Thoughts on narcissism and narcissistic rage. Psychoanal Study Child 27:360–400, 1972

Kohut H: The Restoration of the Self. New York, International Universities Press, 1977

Kohut H: How Does Analysis Cure? Chicago, IL, University of Chicago Press, 1984

Lichtenberg J: Continuities and transformations between infancy and adolescence. Adolesc Psychiatry 10:182–198, 1982

Lichtenberg J: Psychoanalysis and Infant Research. Hillsdale, NJ, Analytic Press, 1983

Lichtenberg J: Psychoanalysis and Motivation. Hillsdale, NJ, Analytic Press, 1989

Marohn D: The "juvenile imposter": some thoughts on narcissism and the delinquent. Adolesc Psychiatry 5:186–212, 1977

Masterson J: Psychotherapy of the adolescent: a comparison with psychotherapy of the adult. J Nerv Ment Dis 127:511–517, 1958

Masterson J: The Psychiatric Dilemma of Adolescence. Boston, MA, Little, Brown, 1967

Masterson J: Treatment of the Borderline Adolescent: A Developmental Approach. New York, Wiley-Interscience, 1972

Meeks J: The Fragile Alliance. Baltimore, MD, Williams & Wilkins, 1971

Miller D: The Age Between: Adolescence and Psychotherapy. New York, Jason Aronson, 1983

Offer D, Offer J: From Teenage to Young Manhood: A Psychological Study. New York, Basic Books, 1975

Piaget J, Inhelder B: The Psychology of the Child. New York, Basic Books, 1969

Rakoff V: The emergence of the adolescent patient. Adolesc Psychiatry 16:372–386, 1989

Schafer R: A New Language for Psychoanalysis. New Haven, CT, Yale University Press, 1976

Schafer R: The Analytic Attitude. New York, Basic Books, 1983

Sklansky M: The alchemy of love: the transmutation of the elements in adolescents and young adults. Annual of Psychoanalysis 5:77–103, 1977

Stern D: The Interpersonal World of the Infant. New York, Basic Books, 1985

Wolf E: Tomorrow's self: Heinz Kohut's contributions to adolescent psychiatry. Adolesc Psychiatry 8:41–50, 1980

Wolf E: Adolescence: psychology of the self and self-objects. Adolesc Psychiatry 10:171–181, 1982

Wolf E, Gedo J, Terman D: On the adolescent process as a transformation of the self. Journal of Youth and Adolescence 1:257–272, 1972

Chapter 3

Biological Facets of Psychotherapy

DEWLEEN G. BAKER, M.D.
KATHLEEN J. HART, Ph.D.

Chapter 3

Biological Facets of Psychotherapy

Most adolescents reach adulthood without having incurred a psychiatric referral. A smooth unfolding of personal experiences and brain development allows teens to mature without major emotional mishap, confident and capable of assuming adult social roles. When this process goes awry, the causes are often complex, reflecting the interacting biological, psychological, and environmental facets of growth and development.

In the evaluation of an adolescent, one may encounter subjective distress expressed by the child, behavioral problems noted by the parents, and difficulties in intrafamilial and interpersonal relationships described by both. Evaluators must appreciate the presenting problem, discern the factors that cause or contribute to the distress, and then devise a plan of treatment. In doing this, knowledge of the role of biological factors is essential.

In this chapter learning disabilities and mood disorders are presented as illustrative examples of these interacting facets. Learning disabilities are approached from the viewpoint of neural development that predisposes adolescents to academic deficiencies, which in turn contribute to social-emotional impairment. Because cognitive abilities mediate the process of psychotherapy, the impact of these deficiencies on such treatment is considerable. The discussion of mood disorders addresses the impact of neurodevelopmental and psychopharmacological correlates to therapy.

For heuristic reasons the two disorders will be discussed separately; however, it should be understood that adolescents with one such psychiatric disorder may, in fact, have another. (A third disorder in which biological factors are prominent, attention-deficit disorder, will be addressed by R. L. Hendren in Chapter 7.)

Learning Disabilities

Although the specific etiology of learning disabilities is unknown, various causes have been proposed. These include prenatal and neonatal medical conditions, such as infection, mild encephalitis, and subtle metabolic disorders, as well as subtle cerebral malformations and immaturities, such as arrested myelination and improperly directed regrowth of severed axons (Rourke et al. 1983). Although numerous causes may be involved, it is generally agreed that the etiology lies within the neurological substrate.

Estimates suggest that 10% to 16% of school-age children experience learning difficulties of sufficient magnitude so as to be labeled "learning disabled." Because the underlying cognitive deficits of this population predispose it to academic, social, or behavioral difficulties, families of the learning disabled often seek psychiatric help. We first present the issues that clinicians treating learning-disabled adolescents typically encounter and discuss their impact on psychotherapy.

Defining Learning Disabilities

The term *learning disability* describes a heterogeneous group of disorders that affect the academic progress of children and adolescents. Given the breadth of disorders encompassed in this single term, a diagnosis of learning disability conveys only the fact that the individual experiences academic difficulties. Not surprisingly, the lack of specificity has engendered much confusion among those who interact with these adolescents. Although there have been several attempts to describe "subtypes" and classification systems, these have not yet met the rigors of systematic evaluation. As such, any subtypes are best considered as hypotheses awaiting empirical study and support (Morris 1988).

In addition to representing an academic and clinical entity, learning disabilities are associated with a strong sociopolitical force that is aimed at making special education services available to children with various handicapping conditions. This force was fueled by the passage of the Education for All Handicapped Children Act (U.S. PL 94-142) in 1975. Although the definition of learning disabilities provided in this act has been subject to widespread criticism, it currently remains the accepted legal definition and serves as the basis for most service delivery policies:

> Specific learning disability means a disorder in one of the basic psychological processes involved in using or understanding language, spoken or written, which may manifest itself in an impaired ability to listen, speak, write, spell, or to do mathematical calculations. The term includes such conditions as perceptual handicaps, brain injury, minimal brain dysfunction, dyslexia, and developmental aphasia. The term does not include children who have learning problems which are primarily the result of visual, hearing, or motor handicaps, mental retardation, emotional disturbance or environmental, cultural or economic disadvantage. (Education for all Handicapped Children Act 1975)

A major focus of this definition is to distinguish "specific" learning disabilities from "general" learning disabilities. Adolescents in the former category typically have average overall intelligence quotients. Because of discrete cognitive deficits, however, their academic performance is below average. In contrast, those in the latter category have limited mental abilities that affect all areas of learning. If clinicians are to successfully intervene on behalf of learning-disabled patients, they must be familiar with this legislation and with the legal and political issues involved.

Assessment Issues and Their Impact on Psychotherapy

Although many learning disabilities are diagnosed during childhood, children may often remain undiagnosed into adolescence. Further, many learning disabilities persist into adolescence and beyond, such that ongoing assessment of previously identified disorders can be helpful in understanding the current impact of the disorder on the adolescent.

Clinicians who suspect learning disabilities must ask two questions when referring such youngsters for educational evaluation: Are specific cognitive deficits having a negative impact on school performance, and are special education services required in order to improve academic performance? Impaired cognitive functioning encompasses the inability to grasp the complexity of social situations, thereby making assimilation into peer groups difficult. Many learning-disabled adolescents suffer the stigma of placement in special classrooms, as well as the cumulative effects of school difficulty. Although research findings suggest that the adjustment of learning-disabled students is highly variable, vulnerabilities of self-esteem are frequently a major psychological issue (Rourke et al. 1983). Also, family dynamics can interact with the learning-disabled student's overall level of adjustment. Parents are concerned about the degree of responsibility the adolescent can assume for behavior and academic performance, and their responses to these issues vary according to the exact nature of their child's disability. Regardless of the particular situation, however, reassurance, support, and education are all critical treatment components.

The following cases shed further light on these issues:

Case 1

Jamie was 13 years old when he was seen for consultation. His parents reported a long history of poor attention, poor academic progress, behavior problems, and diminished self-esteem. They were ambivalent about holding him responsible for many of his actions, and they were worried that their expectations for him were too high. His behavior problems were bringing him in contact with legal authorities, and his parents were discouraged by his poor response to previous psychiatric intervention. He had little insight into his own behavior.

Psychological assessment found Jamie to be a young man of generally high average intelligence. His test scores indicated that his ability to reflect upon and relate his emotional experiences was relatively poor. Placement within a special education program was recommended.

In keeping with Jamie's impulsive behavior and poorly developed verbal facility, the psychiatrist recommended that treatment assume a strong behavioral orientation, rather than a traditional, insight-oriented psychotherapeutic approach. It was felt that this type of approach would enable Jamie to better understand the relationship between behaviors and their consequences. In an effort to strengthen his verbal reasoning skills, problem-solving techniques were incorporated into psychotherapy. A meeting was held with the parents in order to help them view their son as a potentially responsible person and provide them with appropriate disciplinary guidelines. It was hoped that this multifaceted treatment would eventually effect a more positive self-image.

Case 2

Michelle was a 14-year-old eighth-grader when seen for psychiatric consultation. She had few friends and was described by her mother as socially awkward. Since early childhood she had been treated by an ophthalmologist for what her mother termed a "lazy eye." While other developmental milestones had been met within normal limits, Michelle's fine-motor skills had developed slowly and continued to be poor. Early school progress was slow, and school evaluation completed in the third grade concluded that Michelle had a "visual-auditory-perceptual" problem. Special education services were initiated at that time. Because of dramatic improvement in Michelle's academic performance, however, these services were eventually discontinued. When she reached the seventh grade, her grades dropped and she was again evaluated for special education services. Reports indicated that a lack of motivation, rather than a learning disability, accounted for her academic difficulties. Eager to have Michelle qualify for school education services, her parents sought independent evaluation.

When Michelle was seen by the psychiatrist, her behavior was striking. She spoke in an overly familiar and flippant manner, and made many cryptic comments. She was referred to a psychologist, who made similar observations. On several occasions when having made errors during testing, Michelle asserted that the tests were being incorrectly administered. Test results showed that attention and concentration were below average, as were her fine-motor skills. Her ability to organize information spontaneously, maintain a problem-solving set, and demonstrate self-regulation were also well below average.

Michelle was seen in individual psychotherapy, with the aim of improving her social interactions and interpersonal problem-solving skills. The therapy took a directive approach. Michelle was instructed in social conversation and given feedback regarding her performance. Therapy focused on interpreting cues given by others (e.g., "body language" and tone of voice) and on interpersonal problem-solving strategies.

After approximately 6 months of weekly therapy sessions, Michelle began to initiate and maintain friendships. Her newly developed verbal skills enabled her to reflect upon her experiences and feelings. As therapy progressed, she not only was able to articulate her disappointment about rejection by peers but also was able to recognize changes in peers' responses as her own style of interaction changed. Consequently, her self-image gradually improved and she felt more comfortable at school. These factors, in turn, had a positive impact on her academic growth.

In both cases recognition of cognitive disabilities in adolescents led to a treatment approach in which specific behavioral techniques aimed at remediating these disabilities were incorporated. Helping these adolescents develop new problem-solving skills and assisting them with recognizing social cues resulted in enhanced competence and improved self-esteem.

Mood Disorders

A decade ago, the existence of adolescent mood disorders was controversial. The ensuing years have witnessed the development of reliable and valid semistructured interview techniques and operational diagnostic criteria that have paved the way toward systematic research (Puig-Antich 1987). Data now indicate that major depression presents in adolescents in a manner similar to that found in adult populations (Mitchell et al. 1988; Ryan et al. 1987). There are, however, some differences in symptoms and behaviors between adolescents and other age groups. Adolescents acknowledge more hopelessness, helplessness, hypersomnia, and weight changes. They also make more serious suicide attempts than both children and adults (Carlson and Strober 1979; Ryan et al. 1987).

Depressed adolescents are more likely to report hallucinations than are adults. Auditory hallucinations are, in fact, experienced by 10% to 22% of this population. In contrast, adolescents are less likely to experience delusions (Mitchell et al. 1988; Strober et al. 1981).

As with follow-up studies of depressed adults, those studies involving adolescents with affective illnesses attest to the continuity of morbidity over time (Garber et al. 1988; Kandel and Davies 1986). Symptoms of depression in adolescence are the forerunner of similar problems in adulthood, and adolescent dysphoria is generally associated with later difficulties in social functioning (Kovacs et al. 1984).

In contrast to adults, adolescents are more likely to develop a bipolar illness following a depressive episode. One significant study revealed that 20% of adolescents who were initially diagnosed with major depression were diagnosed as having bipolar illness 4 years later (Strober and Carlson 1988). Mixed bipolar disorder, rapid cycling, and hypomania have also been found to occur frequently in adolescents (Puig-Antich 1987). Studies also suggest that bipolar disorder does not always manifest with typical manic episodes in adolescents (Ballenger et al. 1982).

The diagnostic process in adolescents is often complicated by the occurrence of additional disorders (Mitchell et al. 1988). Anxiety and conduct disorders, attention-deficit disorder, eating disorders, learning disabilities, and substance abuse frequently present concurrently. These disorders may alter the severity and/or frequency of symptoms of the mood disorder. Data pertaining to the phenomenology of depression indicate that adolescents with coexisting disorders have a higher mean depression severity than do those with a single diagnosis of depression (Mitchell et al. 1988). Comorbidity of the disorders cited earlier also appears to be a common risk factor for adolescent suicide (Brent et al. 1988).

Neurodevelopmental and Psychopharmacological Factors

The development of neurotransmitter systems begins in the first trimester of gestation. This process continues through late adolescence and on into adult life (Popper 1987). Various anatomical regions and neurotransmitter systems develop at different rates and mature at different times. The psychological and neurophysiological functions that these pathways subserve also change during the course of development. This process results in age-related pharmacodynamic differences in drug responses. These responses may manifest as differences in drug sensitivity or responsivity. The relatively poor response of adolescents and young adults to tricyclic antidepressant therapy appears to be a result of pharmacodynamic factors rather than pharmacokinetic factors (Ryan et al. 1986).

Although pharmacokinetic factors do not appear to be the cause of poorer response rate of adolescents to these medications, these factors are important when considering appropriate dosages. Adolescents may require larger doses of drugs than do adults in order to achieve comparable blood levels. Increased hepatic metabolism is accepted as the major mechanism for this physiological process. Because the time of the change to an adult metabolism that diminishes hepatic activity is variable, 1) frequent measurement of plasma levels, 2) careful clinical monitoring, and 3) flexible dosage adjustment are indicated (Teicher and Baldessarini 1987).

The pharmacokinetics of lithium differ from those of tricyclics in that lithium is excreted by the kidneys. Because renal excretion does not vary dramatically with age, the dosage and monitoring requirements for adolescents are similar to those for adults.

Drug-Related Consideration

Prior to initiating drug treatment, a general medical examination should be obtained. Blood pressure, pulse, height, and weight should be documented, for these parameters are frequently affected by psychotropic medication. When antidepressants are prescribed, base-line and repeated electrocardiograms during dose elevation are necessary to follow cardiac side effects. When lithium is prescribed, a base line of electrolytes, thyroid function studies, and blood creatinine monitoring are indicated. Blood lithium levels are required at least monthly. Blood creatinine levels are required every 3 months to monitor kidney function. Thyroid-stimulating hormone levels may be drawn once or twice a year.

For adolescents receiving long-term psychotropic treatment, height, weight, blood pressure, pulse, tics, and dyskinesias should be documented every 3 to 6 months, and a complete physical examination with routine blood tests should be carried out yearly (Popper 1985).

After medication is begun, comprehensive follow-up is essential. Information on dosage regimens, side effects, and blood levels should be obtained (Robson 1987; Wiener 1987). Treatment records should include target symptoms, the rationale for the drug selection, initial dosages and medication plans, and increases of dosages and responses to these increases. The occurrence of any adverse reactions should also be noted, as should a rationale for changing or discontinuing any medication (Robson 1987). Discussions with adolescents and their parents pertaining to informed consent issues should also be documented.

The following cases highlight the issues involved in prescribing medication:

> Sarah, aged 16, was depressed. Her feelings of hopelessness had led to occasional thoughts of suicide. She was inattentive and sometimes had difficulty falling asleep. She came from an upwardly mobile family who had high aspirations for their children. Sarah's depressive feelings centered around her concern over fulfilling those shared aspirations.

Treatment recommendations included antidepressant medication to ameliorate the depressive symptoms and individual psychotherapy to address the apprehension she felt in living up to her parental ideals. After 4 weeks she was markedly less depressed, was sleeping better, and was less hopeless. She became optimistic about her future and discussed her fears of not living up to her parents' expectations.

John, a 17-year-old high school senior, was brought to outpatient therapy by his parents. They were concerned about depressive symptoms including dysphoria, angry outbursts, crying spells, sleep disturbance, difficulty with concentration, and feelings of hopelessness. Prior to the onset of the symptoms, both John and his parents described their relationship as very good. John was now angry at being coerced into seeing a psychiatrist, and initially refused to speak. When he began to talk, he dated the onset of depressive feelings to the beginning of the school year, when he had broken up with a girlfriend.

Treatment recommendations for antidepressant medication in conjunction with individual psychotherapy brought about an outburst from John. When he stated that he refused to come to another session if he had to take medication, the psychiatrist told John that this decision would be his to make.

Over the next 3 weeks John came to treatment but refused medication. The therapist noted that she respected John's need for independence and autonomy, and continued to inform him of the benefits of the medication. Eventually John agreed to take the antidepressant medication and sustained resolution of his depressive symptoms. At that point he began to discuss with his therapist the precipitant of his depression: the devastating impact of losing his girlfriend.

The two cases illustrate the combined use of medication and individual psychotherapy. In both, the severity of the depressive symptoms accompanied by neurovegetative signs and symptoms led to the initiation of antidepressant treatment. Developing an alliance with the adolescent with shared goals set the stage for agreement of medication use.

Summary

The recognition of the contribution of biological factors to adolescent mental health necessitates a broadened view of psychotherapy. Learning-disabled adolescents require therapists to appreciate the effect of cognitive difficulties on these patients' life experiences and to modify their approach to treatment. Treatment of adolescents with mood disorders encompasses appreciation of both developmental and pharmacological issues.

References

Ballenger JC, Reus VI, Post RM: The "atypical" clinical picture of adolescent mania. Am J Psychiatry 139:602–606, 1982

Brent DA, Perper JA, Goldstein CE, et al: Risk factors for adolescent suicide. Arch Gen Psychiatry 45:581–588, 1988

Carlson GA, Strober M: Affective disorders in adolescent suicide. Psychiatr Clin North Am 2:511–526, 1979

Education for All Handicapped Children Act, PL 94-142, 1, 89, Stat. 773, 20 USCS 1401, 1975

Garber J, Kriss MR, Koch M, et al: Recurrent depression in adolescents: a follow-up study. J Am Acad Child Adolesc Psychiatry 27:49–54, 1988

Kandel DB, Davies M: Adult sequelae of adolescent depressive symptoms. Arch Gen Psychiatry 43:255–262, 1986

Kovacs M, Feinberg TL, Crouse-Novak M, et al: Depressive disorders in childhood, II: A longitudinal study of the risk for a subsequent major depression. Arch Gen Psychiatry 41:643–649, 1984

Mitchell J, McCauley E, Burke PM, et al: Phenomenology of depression in children and adolescents. J Am Acad Child Adolesc Psychiatry 27:12–20, 1988

Morris RD: Classification of learning disabilities: old problems and new approach. J Consult Clin Psychol 56:789–794, 1988

Popper CW: Child and adolescent psychopharmacology, in Psychiatry, Vol 2. Edited by Michaels R, et al. Philadelphia, PA, JB Lippincott, 1985, pp 1–23

Popper C: Medical unknowns and ethical consent: prescribing psychotropic medications for children in the face of uncertainty, in Psychiatric Pharmacosciences of Children and Adolescents. Edited by Popper C. Washington, DC, American Psychiatric Press, 1987, pp 125–161

Puig-Antich J: Affective disorders in children and adolescents: diagnostic validity and psychobiology, in Psychopharmacology: The Third Generation of Progress. Edited by Meltzer HY. New York, Raven Press, 1987, pp 843–859

Robson K (ed): Manual of Clinical Child Psychiatry. Washington, DC, American Psychiatric Press, 1987

Rourke BP: Socioemotional disturbances of learning disabilities: old problems and new approaches. J Consult Clin Psychol 56:789–794, 1988

Rourke BP, Bakker DJ, Fisk JL, et al: Child Neuropsychology: An Introduction to Theory, Research, and Clinical Practice. New York, Guilford, 1983

Ryan ND, Puig-Antich J, Cooper T, et al: Imipramine in adolescent major depression: plasma level and clinical response. Acta Psychiatr Scand 73:275–288, 1986

Ryan ND, Puig-Antich J, Ambrosini P, et al: The clinical picture of major depression in children and adolescents. Arch Gen Psychiatry 44:854–861, 1987

Strober M, Carlson G: Bipolar illness in adolescents with major depression. Arch Gen Psychiatry 27:751–754, 1988

Strober M, Green J, Carlson G, et al: Phenomenology and subtypes of major depressive disorder in adolescence. J Affective Disord 3:281–290, 1981

Teicher MH, Baldessarini RJ: Developmental pharmacodynamics, in Psychiatric Pharmacosciences of Children and Adolescents. Edited by Popper C. Washington, DC, American Psychiatric Press, 1987, pp 45–80

Wiener JM (ed): Diagnosis and Psychopharmacology of Childhood and Adolescent Disorders. New York, John Wiley, 1987

Chapter 4

Social Systems Contributions to Psychotherapy

GLEN T. PEARSON, JR., M.D.

Chapter 4

Social Systems Contributions to Psychotherapy

*T*oday's adolescent struggles for survival and growth in a dynamic, complex, and often chaotic social milieu. Technological developments, particularly in transportation and communication, have combined with fluctuating economic conditions and an increasing diversity of social values to produce an American society that is almost incomprehensibly heterogeneous.

The same geographic and social mobility that provides greater opportunity for wage earners may produce for their children a climate of rootless uncertainty. Economic conditions make it increasingly likely that both parents will be wage earners. Marriages are increasingly likely to end in divorce, and the children of both single-parent and two–wage-earner households are likely to experience less availability of parental nurturance, guidance, and discipline. At the same time, extended family members are less available to adolescents as those to whom they can turn when they are turning away (as they must) from their parents.

The electronic age has provided a generation of adolescents with television as a substitute for individualized caregiving during their preadolescent years. Besides regularly witnessing explicit depictions of acts of violence and of normal and perverse sexuality, children brought up by television enter adolescence with a strongly reinforced sense of entitlement to passive gratification of wishes, wants, and needs, and without a clear sense of differentiation among these (Miller 1983).

Underlying the disparate elements of an increasingly fragmented social system is a broad-based increased emphasis on the rights, needs, and wishes of the individual. This apparent global rise in narcissism on the societal scale (Rinsley 1982) is reflected in such media-popularized phrases as "The 'Me' Generation," "The Sexual Revolution," and "If it feels good, do it." The normative proclivity of the adolescent for preoccupation with self, sex, feeling good, and action, even under the most constricting of conditions, is irrepressibly reinforced by the prevailing social milieu.

Chaotic though it may appear, society encompasses an array of smaller social systems, each of which is governed by its own set of rules. To some extent, the apparent chaos in the larger society can be understood in terms of the diversity of goals and values espoused by the smaller systems, and the perplexity and confusion of some individuals by their simultaneous membership in two or more systems with divergent social values. Individual conflicts associated with multisystem membership are characteristic of the adolescent developmental phase, when, to use a common example, the child may first choose memberships in peer groups whose values may conflict with those of his or her family.

Therapy is not conducted in a vacuum. The adolescent patient comes into the consulting room embedded, as it were, in a nexus of involvement with a variety of social systems in which he or she has membership. These systems have impacted the course of the youngster's development and continue to exert dynamic influence on his or her current life and clinical presentation. Today's adolescents are unavoidably assigned membership in their own family, ethnic group, socioeconomic class, school, and society as a whole. With each passing year of development during adolescence proper, memberships in other social systems become available to teenagers, who choose some by virtue of their inclinations and have others thrust upon them because of their behavior or experiences. Each social system has its own set of rules that govern the interaction among the adolescent and the other members of the system (Haley 1968; Jones et al. 1989); therefore, the therapist's awareness of the patient's systems involvements, and knowledge of the rules of interaction in those systems, are crucial to the therapist's ability truly to understand and help the patient.

An adolescent's psychotherapist must both observe and participate with the patient in the context of the youngster's social systems, which frequently make demands upon both the adolescent and the therapist during the course of treatment. Therapeutic effectiveness is maximized when the therapist can join helpfully not only with the adolescent patient but also with family, school, and community systems in order to facilitate both the development of the adolescent toward healthy functioning as an individual and a more adaptive adjustment to the real world of his or her social environment.

In this chapter I consider the adolescent patient as a member of some of the more important social systems impacting youth (family, school, and community) and propose principles and guidelines for therapists' interactions with adolescents and their social systems.

Systems Theory and Adolescent Psychotherapy

As human beings we experience membership in a variety of social systems throughout the life cycle, beginning with the closed system of symbiotic dual unity shared by infant and mother, and proceeding through progressive levels of differentiation and organization both psychologically and socially. A child's growth and development from infancy through the preschool years take place in the context of a relatively circumscribed social system, the family. Having established the family as a secure base of social operation, school-age children can go on to assume additional memberships in classroom, peer groups, and some organized activities under adult supervision. Adult life is characterized by building, maintaining, and participating in a variety of social systems: one's own relationships, marriage, family, employment, commitments to ideals and organizations, and participation in leisure pursuits with others of like interests.

In the realm of social systems interaction, as in many other functional areas, adolescence is at once ripe with opportunities and fraught with vulnerabilities. The pubertal child must simultaneously cope with an inner explosion of instinctual energies (and the related reactivation of previously dormant conflicts) and a geometrically expanding variety of social systems on the outer horizon. At the same time, adolescents whose problems have necessitated referral for psychotherapy are quite likely to have begun to experience their own family as alien, their parents as wrongheaded and oppressive, and their parents' values as outmoded and inimical to their autonomy. Social systems outside the family provide the adolescent with opportunities to experiment with roles, establish intimate relationships, and work through dependency ties—in short, to proceed with the "second separation-individuation" (Blos 1967) and the establishment of identity (Erikson 1963) that are the hallmarks of developmental success in adolescence.

General systems theory offers the psychotherapist a framework for understanding the adolescent patient's individual issues in the context of his or her involvement in social systems. Systems theory proposes a world made up of systems, hierarchically arrayed and characterized by similarity of underlying structure (isomorphy) and of organizing processes at all levels. Systems are related to each other both vertically (hierarchically) and horizontally (laterally) through the exchange of matter-energy and information at their boundaries, carrying out through these activities three primary system functions: to maintain wholeness, to achieve self-regulation in the face of environmental disturbances, and to achieve progressive self-transformation to higher levels of adaptation (Durkin 1981a). Boundaries are a crucial property of systems of all kinds; it is through selective opening and closing of boundaries that a system interacts with the environment, accomplishes its functions, and constantly reshapes and redefines itself.

Living systems encompass a hierarchy of progressively differentiated and complex subsystems from cell to society. The isomorphic structure of living systems is autonomous (Durkin 1981b); that is, each system regulates its functions from within itself by opening, closing, expanding, or retracting its boundaries. Activity at the boundary is the key process in system functioning, and attempts to influence a system must therefore refer to the boundary. Astrachan (1970), for example, has defined the role of the psychotherapy group leader as primarily one of moderating the boundaries.

An important means by which human social systems establish and regulate boundaries is the evolution of rules that dictate the process of interaction among the members of the system (Bateson et al. 1968). Written examples of these rules abound in history, law, and government; unwritten, and often unacknowledged, rules also govern the interactions among members of families and among other important small groups. The unwritten rules of interaction in social systems are so pervasive that any attempt to influence a system must take account of its rules, just as it does of the boundaries.

The symptomatic behavior that is the focus of therapeutic scrutiny and intervention does not arise solely from within the adolescent. It is a product of the interaction between the adolescent and one or more of the important social systems of which he or she is currently a member. A minimally adequate formulation of the patient's symptoms therefore requires the therapist to attend to the issue of the patient's systems memberships, to acquire a working knowledge of the boundaries and the rules of interaction of each relevant system, and to be aware of how the different systems interface with each other. The successful establishment of a therapeutic relationship with the adolescent creates yet another social system, one in which both the youngster and the therapist are members, and which has significant interface with at least some of the adolescent's other systems. The therapeutic relationship itself, with its boundaries and rules of interaction, must also be considered within the hierarchy of the patient's social world.

The key to understanding systems issues in adolescent psychotherapy is at once simple and metapsychological. It is simple because one must simply remember to "think systems"—to approach the patient bearing in mind his or her possible systems memberships. It is metapsychological because one must then clarify the meaning of the patient's material in the context of his or her memberships in systems, and each system's boundaries and interface with the patient's other systems should be explored and their rules of interaction sketched in detail proportional to their relative impact upon those psychopathological issues that are under consideration.

Sources of Data

In the quest for understanding of the adolescent's world of social relationships, several sources of data are available to the psychotherapist. In most (if not all) cases, initial therapeutic contacts involve meetings with parents. These meetings provide the therapist with an opportunity to experience direct interaction with important members of one of the adolescent's most important social systems, the family. Impressions gleaned from these meetings can be used in individual sessions with the adolescent as a departure point for clarification of the patient's experience as a family member and for obtaining information about the family's unwritten rules of interaction.

> **Patient:** My dad was on his high horse again last night. He thinks he knows everything. If I disagree with him I must be wrong. He was trying to tell me I had no right to be angry because I didn't understand the situation. My mom just sat there giving me looks like, "Be quiet, don't aggravate him."

> **Therapist:** I noticed the same kind of thing happening when I met with you and your parents at the beginning of your therapy. I wonder if one of the rules in your family is that your mom has to keep peace by keeping quiet and trying to keep you quiet too.

Telephone and other contacts with the adolescent's parents, which inevitably occur in the course of treatment, are ongoing sources of data on the family system, which can be clarified, on appropriate occasions, in relation to material brought by the patient.

Another potential source of information concerning the adolescent's social systems is the therapist's own knowledge of, or involvement in, those systems, independent of the therapeutic relationship. Many patients share certain large-system memberships with their therapists, such as socioeconomic class, religious affiliation, or citizenship in a town. If a therapist has seen a number of other children enrolled in a patient's school, he or she may already have at his or her disposal a data base on the patient's school system; the same may be true for other community systems such as churches, youth service agencies, or even particular neighborhoods. As it emerges in the course of treatment that the youngster's involvement in one of these systems may be a factor in the maintenance of his or her psychopathology, the therapist's knowledge of the system in question can be very helpful in formulating interventions. When making use of one's preexisting data base, however, it is important not to presume that the patient has experienced the system in exactly the same way as the therapist, or as his or her other "informants." Careful clarification of the patient's experience of membership in the social system under consideration, explicitly compared with the therapist's data base for congruence, may permit the therapist to use his or her prior knowledge in ways that will increase the patient's feeling of being understood:

> **Patient:** You'd think by the time I'm a sophomore I could have figured out which group of kids I belong with. I just don't seem to fit in with any of them. I don't think anybody likes me.

Therapist: Some kids who used to go to your school told me the kids divided themselves into groups like preppies, head-bangers, punks, and freaks. Is that still the way it is?

Clarification and comparison also provide a safeguard against inappropriate countertransference identification with the patient (in which, for example, one presumes that the patient's experience of membership in a strict religious denomination is identical to the therapist's own past experience in the same denomination), as well as against interventions that are wide of the mark because they are based on data from sources other than the patient.

The adolescent patient himself or herself is the source of most of the data a therapist will get concerning the social systems involvements of the patient. The therapist should listen with a "fourth ear" attuned to possible social systems implications and should pursue those implications via confrontation and clarification as they appear relevant. Social systems with which the therapist has no experience should be made a focus of psychoeducational attention for the therapist. The adolescent can be explicitly cast in a teaching role for this purpose, and most youngsters relish the opportunity to be an "expert":

Patient: You'd have to see it to believe how mean the popular kids at my school are to everybody who's not in their little clique.

Therapist: Well, I haven't seen it, but I think it's an important thing for me to understand. Can you explain more about it to me?

Principles of Involvement

The coming together of an adolescent patient and his or her psychotherapist creates a new social system, a therapeutic dyad, in which the therapist has the advantage of being able to define the boundaries and rules of interaction rather than simply letting them evolve. Each therapist has ground rules for therapy that spring from a complex combination of training, theoretical orientation, and personal style; each therapist orients his patients to these rules of interaction. Within the boundaries of the therapeutic dyad, the therapist should address issues of the adolescent's functioning in social systems outside the therapy as the relevance of those systems becomes clear in the course of treatment. If this type of psychotherapeutic intervention is effective, the adolescent either may reach a higher level of adaptation to the extratherapeutic systems or may himself or herself become the agent of beneficial adjustments in those systems.

However, the therapeutic dyad is seldom, if ever, insulated from interface with at least some of the adolescent's other systems. The dyad has interfaced from the beginning with the patient's family system because of the patient's membership in both systems and because of the therapist's contractual relationship with the parents (or other adults legally responsible for the adolescent's care). It is therefore incumbent on the therapist to define the boundary and the rules for interaction between the therapeutic system and the family system. In order to do this, one must first be clear about the purpose of the interaction and then promulgate the rules in the light of a few simple principles.

Therapists commonly interact with adolescents' parents with three rather straightforward purposes: evaluation, contracting, and information sharing. In these interactions the parents and the therapist are working together to establish or maintain a system of support for the adolescent's therapy, and the focus of intervention remains within the dyadic relationship. A fourth purpose of interaction with the family system, intervention, aims at making changes in the family system, either by addressing family dysfunction or by making adjustments that one thinks will benefit the adolescent. This is a very different matter from the interactions of contracting, evaluation, and information sharing, which are incidental to any episode of psychotherapy with an adolescent. The rules of interaction among therapist, patient, and family will be defined differently if the family is to be the focus of intervention, and an optimal individual therapeutic relationship with the adolescent may be precluded by those rules. For this reason, careful clarification of the purpose of therapist interaction with the family is essential. If it appears that intervention in the family is to be one of the purposes of interaction, a colleague should be consulted to be the family's therapist. The rules defined for the interaction would then involve communication between the adolescent's and the family's therapists, as well as contact between the parents and each individual therapist involved.

The principles that govern the interaction between the therapist and the family system should also govern the therapist's interaction with any other social systems that present themselves in the course of therapy. Although few in number and relatively simple, these principles can be very difficult to follow.

First, assuming that the family shares with the therapist a common goal of helping the adolescent get back on track developmentally, the therapist is contracting not only with the adolescent for therapy but also with the family as well to create a system of support for the work that the therapist and the youngster will be doing together. The therapist, who has been hired by the family for his or her expertise, must have the authority to define the boundaries and the rules of interaction in this system.

Second, therapeutic success for an adolescent depends on the establishment of a unique relationship with his or her therapist. Interactions of third parties and other systems with the adolescent's therapist are often inimical to the preservation of this special relationship. The boundary between the therapeutic system and the family system must be selectively semipermeable. The "rules of interaction" between therapist and parents (and other third parties) flow from this principle: parents may contact the therapist at any time, but should let the patient know about the contact; the therapist should advise the patient of the fact and content of any communication with the parents. The adolescent's privilege of confidentiality is conditioned only by the therapist's duty to notify the parents if their child is placing himself or herself or other persons in danger by his or her behavior.

Third, the therapist should have as little interaction as possible, or as much as necessary, with parents, other third parties, and relevant social systems of the adolescent. Interaction with parents is always necessary for evaluation, information sharing, and contractual matters. If possible, information should be shared between therapist and parents only in the presence of the adolescent; if this is not possible, both parents and patient should have a prior understanding that the therapist will communicate the content received from the parents to the patient. Therapists should be alert to the possibility that repeated requests for information, or contacts concerning billing or payment, may represent disguised bids for therapeutic attention to one or both of the parents, or to the family system itself. This situation may necessitate further contact with the family to evaluate, clarify, and plan treatment for family system dysfunction. If at all possible, such intervention should be undertaken by a professional other than the adolescent's therapist.

In summary, individual therapy can best be conducted within the boundary of the dyadic relationship, providing that the therapist attends to the adolescent's material from the larger perspective of the adolescent's involvement in social systems outside the therapy. The adolescent's family, or those *in loco parentis*, should be invited to contract with the therapist to create a system of support for the therapeutic work. The therapist should define the rules for all interactions with the adolescent's social systems in such a way that the unique therapeutic relationship is preserved (Pearson 1987).

Having outlined the principles that should guide the therapist's understanding of, and involvement with, the adolescent's social systems, we now turn to a consideration of some of the important social systems in which adolescent patients are actually members: family, school, and a variety of social groups, organizations, and agencies in the community.

The Family

The adolescent's family is preeminent among his or her human systems. While an adolescent's therapist may not encounter a need for involvement with other systems, some interaction with the patient's family is inevitable. Attention to the principles of involvement outlined in the foregoing section can simplify the therapist's task of responding appropriately to the increasingly bewildering array of variations in family structure and systems that currently confront the practitioner of adolescent psychotherapy.

At the beginning of the first session of evaluation of an adolescent for psychotherapy, both parents should be interviewed in the presence of the patient. It is best to begin this interview by first explaining to the adolescent how the assessment will proceed:

> **Therapist:** Your parents have some concerns about your behavior that you and I are going to look at together. First, I need to hear from your mom and dad exactly what their concerns are. After they have explained them, you and I will talk alone, and you can give your side of the story.

Parents bringing a child to psychotherapy are usually themselves unprepared for a therapeutic process (Hoffman 1984). By speaking first to the adolescent, the therapist attempts to establish the primacy of the therapist-patient relationship, while conveying to the parents that the therapist will carefully listen to their input and use their data in evaluating and treating their child. In the process of gathering data on the adolescent's history, the therapist can also clarify the parental roles in the family and make some preliminary observations of the family's pattern of communication. These initial observations and impressions of the "rules of inter-action" in the family system can be clarified with data from the patient in private interviews later in the evaluation.

During the initial phase of the therapist's relationship with the adolescent patient, contact with the family is for purposes of evaluation. If the results of the evaluation establish a need for psychotherapy, the therapist should meet again with the parents and the adolescent to report the findings and recommendations, answer questions, and negotiate a contract for treatment. The process of negotiation should establish a sense that the therapist is contracting with the parents for the common purpose of helping their child, while also entering with the adolescent into the individual therapeutic relationship. The "working alliance" with the parents must complement the "therapeutic alliance" with the adolescent (Schimel 1973); both parents and child must be able to trust the therapist, even though they may be unable to trust each other.

The boundaries and rules of interaction between therapist and parents should be clarified in the contract for treatment. Most parents have little difficulty understanding the adolescent's need for confidentiality, at least in principle. Many parents, however, experience considerable difficulty in trusting their child to communicate fully and honestly with the therapist, and a "one-way open line" from parents to therapist (functionally, a selectively permeable boundary) is helpful in allaying the parents' fears. The parents may contact the therapist to share information they think he or she should have, but the therapist may not divulge information that the patient has shared with him or her. The parents are encouraged to tell the patient if they are planning to contact the therapist; whether or not they do, the therapist will. In addition, the therapist may disclose to the patient what the parents have said. On the other hand, the parents should be reassured that if the therapist learns anything from the patient that the parents need to know in order to provide for his or her health or safety (or their own), the therapist will advise them immediately. In practice, this is seldom necessary, and even when the need arises, it can usually be handled by encouraging the patient to tell the parents and then ensuring that this has been done.

If the therapist succeeds in establishing both a working alliance with the parents and a therapeutic alliance with the adolescent, therapy can proceed with a minimum of direct interaction with the family. The adolescent can then use the therapeutic experience to adapt at a higher level to this family system as it is (that is, as the patient and his or her therapist have come to understand it in relation to the patient's own intrapsychic processes), or to initiate adaptational change in the family system itself. The following case history illustrates these points:

> Matt, 17 years old, had been in individual therapy for over a year. During the first few months of his treatment, his parents and older sister had participated with him in family therapy, under the supervision of a colleague of his individual therapist. The suppression of aggressive derivatives was a major issue both in Matt's and in the family's therapeutic processes. Family therapy had been stopped when Matt's sister left home to attend college. Matt had continued working well in therapy, with no further direct contact between his parents and his therapist, until, after a few sessions of hinting that his frustration with his parents was building toward an explosion again, he revealed that he and his parents had in fact regressed to a former, noncommunicative style of interaction:
>
> > **Matt:** I'm 17 years old and my parents still treat me like a baby. I have to turn off my light and be in bed by 10:00 every night. Most nights I'm not even sleepy by 10:00, and I still have a lot of homework to do.
> > **Therapist:** Have you talked to your folks about your feelings about this rule?
> > **Matt:** It wouldn't do any good.
> > **Therapist:** It won't if you don't do it. You know, rules that are right for a 14-year-old aren't the same as for a 17-year-old. We already know that you and your parents don't talk to each other very much. Maybe you grew up to 17 without their noticing. Maybe if you pointed it out to them, without getting angry and explosive, they'd be willing to negotiate with you about it.
>
> Next session, Matt reported that his parents had "compromised" with him: they were willing to let him choose his own bedtime so long as he got up on time in the morning.

Family Systems Issues and Family Configuration

As the 20th century draws, wearily, to a close, it seems increasingly seldom in clinical practice that one encounters an adolescent whose biological parents are still married to each other. The social trends of the past 30 years have resulted in a variety of family constellations that have complicated the family systems issues to which the therapist of adolescents must attend. A few of the more or less commonly seen configurations that the therapist may be called upon to address are described below.

Traditional (two-parent) families. Traditional families are still occasionally encountered in clinical populations of adolescents; however, even intact families are less likely than in the past to conform to the traditional model in which the father is wage earner and disciplinarian, and the mother the homemaker and caregiver of the children. In the evaluation phase of his or her work with the youngster, the therapist should make note of any idiosyncratic ways in which the family has provided for the carrying out of these traditional family tasks. The parents' opinions concerning the child's need for treatment may be different; they may even disagree on the facts of the history. Such disparities should be noted and an attempt made to understand them from the perspective of the ongoing pattern of relationships among parents and child. Nonjudgmental exploration of these differences of opinion often produces much valuable information on the family's interactional style, system flexibility and openness, and overall level of competence (Lewis 1980; Lewis et al. 1976).

Single-parent families. Families in which one (usually divorced) parent has the sole responsibility of child rearing present the adolescent's therapist with what appears to be on the surface a simpler interactional task. In fact, the single-parent family is often more difficult to understand as a system. In the absence of a spouse, to whom does the remaining parent turn for a variety of interdependent needs: love, sex, companionship, partnership in decision making and parenting? To the extent that these needs are directed within the nuclear family, a child, particularly of the opposite sex, may unconsciously become a mate to the parent, resulting in an intensification of the usual reactivation of oedipal wishes in early adolescence, an overwhelming of defenses that are undergoing reorganization, and a regression in the ego manifested by seriously disturbed behavior.

To the extent that the parent's adult interpersonal needs are directed outside the nuclear family, complex boundary problems may ensue. For example, a single mother may turn to her parents for financial support, to her women friends for help with parental decisions, and to a boyfriend for love and companionship. Each of these interactions opens the family system, through the mother, to an interface with the world beyond the family that will ultimately be expressed in an impact upon the adolescent. And each interface is in dynamic flux—none is reified in law or cultural tradition—and all these interfaces may be invisible unless the therapist inquires specifically about them in the evaluation and listens attentively to the patient's material with a fourth, or "systems," ear.

Blended families (or step-families). Blended families in which the custodial parent has remarried present a two-parent constellation with complex systems ramifications. Among adolescents referred for psychotherapy, conflict with a step-parent is a common presenting problem. Children of divorce frequently idealize their absent biological parents, and even when an adolescent consciously denigrates the absent parent, the step-parent is usually resented as well. The dynamics of family interaction become particularly complicated when both partners bring children from previous marriages into the newly blended family. Issues and conflicts long dormant in the natural family are reactivated under the influence of the availability of new objects for rivalry, jealousy, and drive discharge. The psychotherapist treating an adolescent from such a family situation is well advised to keep his scorecard of rivals and allies up-to-date by frequently inquiring into the vicissitudes of the family's life.

The most arduous task of family systems comprehension and interaction falls to the therapist of an adolescent whose parents, though divorced, are both actively involved with the patient. This state of affairs appears to be occurring more frequently in recent years, due, no doubt, to the increasing popularity of "joint custody" divorce decrees. More conventional divorce arrangements also provide for continuation of relationship between the adolescent and the noncustodial parent; and wherever these rights are exercised, the adolescent's therapist must take into account the patient's continuing involvement with both of his or her divorced parents, and their separate family systems. Often, a noncustodial parent is mandated by judicial decree to bear the expense of the child's treatment, thus setting up a situation in which the parent bringing the adolescent to therapy expects the other parent to pay the bill. Such circumstances are ripe for the reactivation of conflict between the ex-spouses, and to the extent (often considerable) to which the adolescent patient is involved in the conflict between his or her divorced parents, the therapist may also experience pressure to become involved. This situation is managed by carefully following the principles of therapist involvement with both divorced parents' family systems. While this can be extraordinarily difficult to do, the additional time and effort spent establishing common cause with both parents, and defining the rules of interaction for them, are essential to securing a stable context for the adolescent's treatment. This procedure will also pay significant dividends in the longer term, such as data for therapy and minimization of parental resistances. The following case history illustrates this situation:

> Michael was 13 years old when he was brought to the therapist by his mother because of school failure, rebellious behavior, and suicidal threats. His parents had been divorced for 4 years, during which time they had returned to court on numerous occasions to modify the terms of a joint custody arrangement that, at the time of referral, found Michael and his older sister living with their mother from precisely 6:00 P.M. each Wednesday until precisely 10:00 A.M. each Sunday, and the remainder of their week with their father. Michael's mother, a self-consciously artistic, demonstrative woman, described the reasons for her divorce from, and continuing conflict with, her ex-husband as an ineluctable struggle between opposites. Michael's father, in her view, was a rigid, compulsive, organized cardiologist whose lack of warmth and availability, combined with excessively high and inflexibly held expectations of academic achievement, was a major factor in Michael's emotional and behavioral symptoms. Furthermore, warned the mother, her ex-husband was hostile to the idea of psychotherapy and would probably have to be taken to court to force him to meet his legal responsibility to pay for Michael's treatment.
>
> As part of the evaluation process, the therapist asked that Michael come twice a week, once during his stay with his mother and once during his dad's portion of the week. In addition to forming an alliance with Michael and evaluating his treatment needs, the therapist spent some time with the parent who brought him, taking additional history, sampling the parent-child relationship process, and sketching the rules of interaction for therapy. Michael's father proved as concerned about his son as was the mother, although for different reasons. By the end of a period of evaluation consisting of six visits, both parents were able to enter with the therapist into separate contracts to support Michael in a course of individual psychotherapy (including, on the father's part, a commitment for payment).

The School

Contemporary urban and suburban secondary schools are complex social systems that serve not only educational but also other, less well-defined social purposes. Their primary mission, broadly defined, is not dissimilar to that of the family: "to prepare the young to become successful adult workers, members of families, and citizens" (Comer 1986). For adolescents the school is not only a workplace but also a locus of intersection of diverse peer and community social groups—a laboratory for experimenting with identity. Psychiatric problems of adolescents are often expressed in either social maladjustment in the school or impaired academic performance; the conflict between teenagers and their parents that is often the proximate cause for referral frequently centers around school behavior. Even in those (relatively uncommon) cases in which the adolescent patient's school adjustment and academic performance are preserved, the youngster's experience of school life will usually figure prominently in the therapeutic material.

Mental health professionals' involvement with school systems can be conceptualized on three levels. First, an adolescent's psychotherapist must always attend to the patient's productions with an awareness of the importance of school-system issues. At this level, therapist "involvement" remains within the dyadic therapeutic relationship. In cases in which academic performance is unaffected and school behavior or adjustment problems are understood as secondary to psychological factors unrelated to school, the therapist may elect to treat these problems as one of the symptoms of the adolescent's psychopathology, as reflected in a generalized problem in adjustment to his or her social systems. The adolescent brings his or her day-to-day life experiences to therapy, and the therapist attempts to help the child by clarifying and interpreting intrapsychic and systems issues. Consequently, no direct contact between therapist and school is necessary.

Another type of therapist involvement with school systems exists on the opposite end of the spectrum: mental health professionals may enter into consultation agreements with the school system, in which the focus of consultant attention is either an identified subgroup of "problem" students or the system itself. In the consultation model of involvement, issues of primary and secondary prevention are addressed, and the consultant's responsibility to the school system precedes any individual psychopathological issues that may be identified in the course of the consultation. Although the consultant may be helpful to individual students via recommendations and referrals, a true psychotherapeutic relationship is precluded by the context of the consultation contract. (A discussion of the conceptual issues involved in school consultation is beyond the scope of this chapter; the interested reader is referred to the work of Comer [1986] and Steinberg and Yule [1985].)

At a third, and intermediate, level of involvement, the therapist makes direct contact with the school system for the purpose either of evaluation and information sharing or of collaborative intervention to help the individual patient. If, for example, academic failure was one of the reasons for referral, one is obligated to investigate, via appropriate individualized assessments, whether learning disabilities or cognitive deficits might be factors in the presenting problem. Some, if not all, of the necessary assessments may have already been conducted by the school or, if not, may be available through the school as part of the educational service to which the patient is entitled. The therapist should request permission of the patient and family to receive this information. Other kinds of information that may need to be shared between therapist and school personnel include classroom teachers' observations on social behavior and learning difficulties, response to medication, and counselors' or principal's observations on the adolescent's relationship to authority, peer relationships, and response to discipline.

At the level of direct therapist-school interaction, one is responding to the needs of adolescents who are significantly impaired in school functioning. Most patients who require this level of interaction in adolescence should be certified by the school system as eligible for special education services. The therapist may be called upon by the school staff to provide information that will allow them to certify the patient's eligibility for special services. Both this designation and the interaction that the therapist undertakes with the school on the adolescent's behalf have serious implications for the adolescent's therapy. Adolescents typically resent and resist anything that marks them out as different from their peers, particularly if inferiority is imputed.

The therapist should initiate contact with the adolescent patient's school only with prior permission from both the adolescent and his or her parents, and with clear indications and objectives. It is better if the initiative for therapist-school contact comes from the patient than if the therapist suggests it. Requests for therapist interaction with school personnel coming from any other quarter (i.e., school staff or parents) must be carefully processed with the patient before taking any action. Once liaison has been established, the principles and rules of therapist interaction with the adolescent's social systems apply: the therapist is contracting with the school to help the adolescent; the adolescent's confidences are respected; the therapist will have as little contact as possible, or as much as necessary, with the school staff. It is immensely helpful in adhering to these rules if a single staff person at school is designated liaison with the therapist. Over time, the therapist and school counselor can develop a working relationship in which appropriate information is shared and consultation given, with the result that the adolescent may begin to experience school as supportive of his or her growth, just as the therapist is.

The Community

The term "community," in contemporary usage, denotes a wide variety of social systems—cities, towns, neighborhoods, and populations within them—stratified by social variables such as race, ethnicity, socioeconomic status, business and professional pursuits, ideological commitments, and even common psychosocial deviations and impairments. Thus, we often speak of the black and Hispanic "communities," the banking community, the psychiatric community, the peace community, the gay or lesbian community, and the "recovering community." These designations appear to reflect a universal wish to recapture through large-systems memberships a sense of belonging and togetherness that for many people has been lost in consequence of the decline of the nuclear and extended families, and related small-system institutions.

Adolescents, for the most part, "inherit" their large-systems memberships (e.g., race, ethnicity, socioeconomic status, neighborhood). These large-scale social systems generally cannot be defined in terms of discrete elements with which the adolescent interacts, yet they exert decisive influences on the youngster's growth, development, and emotional life. Although therapists cannot interact directly with elements of the adolescent's "inherited" social systems, it is crucially important that they understand these systems in terms of the impact they have upon the adolescent and the context that they provide for the youngster's daily living experience.

Other community systems memberships are "acquired" in adolescence. Some of these are chosen by the child (e.g., sports teams, musical organizations, Scouts), and others may be thrust upon the child either because of circumstances beyond his or her control (e.g., welfare, child protective services) or because of his or her own behavior (e.g., juvenile justice or mental health authorities). The community systems in which an adolescent may "acquire" membership, particularly those that are thrust upon him, often demand that the therapist interact directly with other elements of the system. Thus, the role of psychotherapist for adolescent patients must encompass both the knowledge required for understanding the youngsters' "inherited" social systems and the skill required for interacting appropriately with those systems in which their patients have "acquired" membership.

General principles that should be followed by therapists of minority adolescents have been described in a relatively voluminous literature, which has focused more upon black patient–white therapist dyads than on other racial combinations (Griffith 1977). One must actively educate oneself in the culture of the patient, be aware of one's own racial and ethnic prejudices, and facilitate open, frank discussion of racial and ethnic issues in the therapeutic sessions. The therapist must guard against any racially based tendency to over-identify or under-identify with the patient (Brantley 1983). Judicious self-disclosure by the therapist may facilitate the process of establishing optimal therapeutic engagement with minority youth.

Eddie, a 15-year-old black adolescent, was trying to explain to his therapist, a white male, how he felt about his experience in the predominantly upper–middle-class white high school into which he had recently transferred:

> **Eddie:** ... and in that whole school there are only a few black kids. Some of them hang out together, but most of them already have some friends. Either way, they don't want anything to do with me. Nobody's been mean to me, exactly, but nobody really speaks to me, either.
> **Therapist:** You know, Eddie, when I was in high school ... a long time ago, and in a part of the country where black kids weren't allowed to go to school with white kids at all, I used to wonder what it would feel like to be a black kid in a school that was set up just for whites. I decided it would probably feel a lot like what I think you are describing now.

Where attempts to assimilate have resulted in cultural transition because of conflicts between the minority and majority cultures, minority adolescents may have been deprived of the normative opportunity for identification with their parents' religious, social, and cultural values (Berlin 1987). Under those conditions, adolescents experience a heightened sense of anomie. Minority adolescents may use a different vocabulary (Comer 1986), or postulate different values (Carter 1979), from those that the majority espouses. The adolescent's psychotherapist must understand the patient's values and vocabulary, and communicate that understanding to the patient, without feeling compelled either to use the vocabulary or to endorse the values. Therapists should bear in mind Erikson's (1968) caveat: that the effects of racism and discrimination leave the minority adolescent vulnerable to the establishment of a "negative identity." Many minority adolescent patients have a culturally determined expectation of authoritarian behavior by the therapist that is at variance with the usual practice of most psychotherapists (Tsui and Schultz 1985). The therapist should be aware of these liabilities and, if necessary, take active countermeasures.

Ethnic or racial minority status is often, but not always, linked with socioeconomic class. Children of upper–middle-class minority families may bear more resemblance to peers of their economic group than to those of their ethnic heritage, and majority adolescents from poor families tend to present the same constellation of deprivation, school failure, and delinquent behaviors that is commonly associated with minority children of poverty. On the opposite end of the economic spectrum, the teenage children of the extremely wealthy pose their own kinds of problems for therapists: as individuals they may expect that the world will change to suit them rather than their having to adapt to the world; as family members they may receive support for such an idiosyncratic perception. Whether the adolescent is rich or poor, black or white, the therapist's task is the same: to understand the patient from the perspective of the patient's membership in his or her social world and the rules of interaction in that society, and to help the adolescent to reach a higher level of adaptation to his or her social world, and, to the extent possible, to become the agent of beneficial changes in his or her own social systems. In working with adolescents from racial, ethnic, and socioeconomic groups different from their own, therapists must endeavor to "get inside their patients' skin"—a task generically identical to that which confronts the therapist of an adolescent from his or her own racial and socioeconomic class, but more difficult to achieve.

The involvements that adolescents acquire with social service agencies call for skillful handling by the therapist. When child welfare or juvenile justice authorities themselves initiate referral of a youngster to a mental health professional, one must carefully clarify whether the referral is for evaluation or for therapy. Referrals of juveniles for "evaluation" by both juvenile justice and child protective services often involve a presumption that the evaluating professional will provide an opinion, either by written report or by testimony, concerning legal issues affecting disposition of a pending case. In most, if not all, such cases, the obligation to render an informed professional opinion to parties other than the child (and those with whom the child is psychologically involved) is tantamount to a conflict of interest that precludes a psychotherapeutic relationship. If the referral purports to be for "therapy," one is well advised to inquire whether there are any unresolved legal issues whatsoever in the case and, even if reassured to the contrary, to explain to the patient (and those responsible for him or her) that there may be an irresolvable incompatibility between one's role as therapist and any unforeseen requirement that one provide information to the court.

Adolescents who are already engaged in psychotherapy may also become secondarily involved with social service agencies. A child may disclose sexual or physical abuse to the therapist, and the therapist is then obligated to report the allegation of abuse to the child protective service agency. If the therapist is to maintain his or her role as the child's helper, it will be essential that he or she does not become embroiled in the subsequent investigation of the alleged abuse. As therapist, one's task is to help the child understand and integrate his or her life experience, which is a very different matter from the investigator's task of establishing fact.

Adolescent patients may also become involved with juvenile justice officials by virtue of illegal acts that they commit as part of their characteristic pattern of symptomatic behavior. When working with teenagers prone to this kind of behavior, one should advise them at the outset that they, and they alone, are responsible for their behavior, and that rescuing them from the consequences of their behavior is incompatible with the therapist's role. Occasionally, one may be asked to collaborate with a probation officer (or child welfare worker) who is *in loco parentis* for a particular child; in such cases the rules of interaction are defined as if the worker in question were the parent (or responsible family member) in the normative case.

In the broad realm of the "community," therapists of adolescents must be vigilant concerning their roles, responsibilities, and boundaries. Evaluative and fact-finding roles are usually incompatible with therapeutic responsibilities. Mental health professionals working with adolescents who are involved with community service agencies should take care that their patients, and the agencies with which they are involved, understand and respect the limitations imposed on the therapist by his or her role in the circumstances of the case.

Conclusions

The adolescent psychotherapy patient must be considered in the context of his or her membership in a multiplicity of social systems, including family, school, and community systems. The therapist of adolescents incurs an obligation to understand not only the intrapsychic processes that govern the individual's unconscious mental life but also the human systems processes that provide a context for the expression of the individual's unconscious derivatives. As a focus of therapeutic understanding and intervention, the adolescent's involvement in social systems is as important as his or her intrapsychic process. Effective psychotherapy with adolescents requires that the therapist attend both to the intrapsychic and to the systems variables of patients' emotional experience and social functioning.

References

Astrachan BM: Towards a social systems model of therapeutic groups. Soc Psychiatry 5:110–119, 1970

Berlin IN: Prevention of psychiatric disorder in American Indian children and adolescents, in Basic Handbook of Child Psychiatry, Vol 5. Edited by Noshpits JD. New York, Basic Books, 1987, pp 600–612

Blos P: The second individuation process of adolescence. Psychoanal Study Child 22:167–186, 1967

Brantley T: Racism and its impact on psychotherapy. Am J Psychiatry 140:1605–1608, 1983

Carter JH: Frequent mistakes made with Black patients in psychotherapy. J Natl Med Assoc 71:1007–1009, 1979

Comer JP: School consultation, in Psychiatry, Vol 2. Edited by Michels R, et al. New York, Basic Books, 1986, pp 1–10

Durkin JE: Foundations of autonomous living structure, in Living Groups: Group Psychotherapy and General Systems Theory. Edited by Durkin J. New York, Brunner/Mazel, 1981a, pp 24–59

Durkin JE: Introduction: the work of the general systems theory committee of the American Group Psychotherapy Association, in Living Groups: Group Psychotherapy and General Systems Theory. Edited by Durkin J. New York, Brunner/Mazel, 1981b, pp xiii–xxvii

Erikson E: Childhood and Society. New York, WW Norton, 1963, pp 247–274

Erikson E: Race and the wider identity, in Identity: Youth and Crisis. New York, WW Norton, 1968, pp 295–320

Griffith MS: The influences of race on the psychotherapeutic relationship. Psychiatry 40:27–40, 1977

Haley J: The family of the schizophrenic: a model system, in Communication, Family and Marriage. Edited by Jackson D. Palo Alto, CA, Science and Behavior Books, 1968, pp 71–199

Hoffman MD: The parents' experience with the child's therapist, in Parenthood: A Psychodynamic Perspective. Edited by Cohen RS, Cohler BJ, Weissman SH. New York, Guilford, 1984, pp 164–172

Jones J, Pearson G, Dimperio R: Long-term treatment of the hospitalized adolescent and his family: an integrated systems-theory approach. Adolesc Psychiatry 16:449–472, 1989

Lewis JM: The family matrix in health and disease, in The Family: Evaluation and Treatment. Edited by Hofling CK, Lewis JM. New York, Brunner/Mazel, 1980, pp 5–44

Lewis JM, Beavers WR, Gossett J: No Single Thread. New York, Brunner/Mazel, 1976

Miller D: The Age Between: Adolescence and Therapy. New York, Jason Aronson, 1983

Pearson GT: Long-term treatment needs of hospitalized adolescents. Adolescent Psychiatry 14:342–357, 1987

Rinsley DB: Borderline and Other Self Disorders. New York, Jason Aronson, 1982

Schimel JL: Two alliances in the treatment of adolescents: toward a working alliance with parents and a therapeutic alliance with the adolescent. J Am Acad Psychoanal 2:243–253, 1973

Steinberg D, Yule W: Consultative work, in Child and Adolescent Psychiatry: Modern Approaches. Edited by Rutter M, Hersov L. Oxford, UK, Blackwell Scientific Publications, 1985, pp 914–926

Tsui P, Schultz G: Failure of rapport: why psychotherapeutic engagement fails in the treatment of Asian clients. Am J Orthopsychiatry 55:561–569, 1985

Treatment

Considerations in the Psychotherapy of Adolescents

ROBERT M. GALATZER-LEVY, M.D., S.C.

Chapter 5

Considerations in the Psychotherapy of Adolescents

An anxious, angry mother telephones about her teenage boy. Despite his "brilliance," he does "miserably in school." She wants a therapist to "do something." In his first session the boy talks reluctantly. Seeing a therapist is another of mother's bids to make him perfect. He just wants to be "ordinary" like his father, whom mother divorced. "Everyone," from his teachers, who "suspect an occult learning disorder," to his step-mother's therapist, who is certain that his salvation is possible only through his mother's analysis, believes that they know what is wrong and what should be done. Who will pay for treatment is disputed between the parents. The youngster's schedule precludes coming to an appointment except on Thursday afternoons at 5:00 P.M., when the therapist is not in the office. The therapist has some ideas about the psychology of the youngster and his family, but is far from able to "do something about it." He does make one recommendation—"Let's talk about it."

As this case so poignantly illustrates, when considering psychotherapy with adolescents, therapists must be aware of the immediate distress experienced by patients, their families, and those around them. Pressure for therapists to "do something" comes from all sides, as well as from within. Ironically, the ever increasing array of possible interventions and fashionable treatments often intensifies their dilemma. The need for a framework that considers these dimensions thus seems apparent.

The Psychotherapeutic Process

The psychotherapeutic process can be conceptualized in terms of its general aims, the nature of the collaboration between therapist and patient, the patient's response to the therapist, the therapist's response to the patient, the goals of treatment, and the process of its termination.

In this chapter I present a framework for incorporating the special aspects of adolescent development into this process. A core tenet of this framework, based on classic psychoanalytic concepts, is that as people become functionally aware of their own psychologies in a context of adequate support, they can reconsider and rework old decisions about how to function.

If the reader comes away with the notion that although work with adolescents is trying, understanding and explanation are often potent tools—then the goal of the chapter will have been achieved.

Principles and Goals of Adolescent Psychotherapy

The general principles of psychotherapy with adolescents are the same as those that govern work with adults. Therapists and patients form an alliance to assist the latter in achieving their own goals. Transferences are appreciated and understood; they are not enacted or exploited, even for therapeutic gain.

The central goal of adolescent psychotherapy is to renew the adolescent's capacity to grow and develop. Health is the ability to engage in further development, not a state from which symptoms are absent (A. Freud 1958/1969; Galatzer-Levy 1988). When treatment goes well, however, youngsters take away even more than the resumption of development. They learn something of how to approach and rectify situations that cause them difficulty later on. This capacity may vary from the largely unconscious ability to rework fantasies and aspects of the personality to simply taking away "words of wisdom" from the therapist (Weiss 1981).

Special Dimensions of Adolescent Psychotherapy

The practice of adolescent psychotherapy is complex. Adolescents are typically brought to treatment either by dissatisfied parents or by school personnel. This situation may lead to confusion on the part of therapists regarding with whom they are allied. Both therapists and patients may view transferences as "realistic" and lose the perspective of understanding as the major activity. Therapists, patients, and families alike may believe that some normative state is to be achieved through treatment. Attempting to enact their own desires and fantasies, parents may put both patient and therapist under enormous pressure. Rather than focusing on resumed growth, therapy may center on a particular achievement that is not of central psychological importance to the patient.

To give an example of what can go awry in this context, we can refer to the youngster mentioned in the opening vignette. Upon being interviewed, it became clear to the psychiatrist that he was depressed. His poor academic performance was a symptom of his depression. It was also evident that the depression was related to the loss of the boy's father. The boy consciously fantasized that had his father remained part of his life, his father would have taught him to be a man. In the transference a strong idealization developed. It seemed pleasant and appropriate for the patient to learn things from his therapist. The transference was understood simply as reflecting a developmental "need" of the patient. The therapist and patient enjoyed their work and the boy's school work improved. From the patient's point of view, however, school work was relatively unimportant: it was something his mother wanted and was unrelated to his own wishes. When the therapist supported the exploration of these feelings, the apparently good situation fell apart. The mother then wanted to stop treatment because the therapist was not doing what she believed he should be doing—improving the boy's grades. The patient had no tools with which to explore his own responses. He viewed the therapist as his mentor. And the therapist was puzzled, since guiding the boy in an exploration of his feelings seemed therapeutically appropriate.

So the intensity of the therapeutic process itself derives from the intensity that adolescents bring into therapy as a result of the myriad of changes they are experiencing and the possible turmoil they are feeling, as well as the intensity of environmental responses and therapists' responses to the adolescents.

Adolescent Changes and Their Impact on Treatment

Physical change. The most obvious changes that take place in adolescents are those that occur in the body and in the experience of the body. The intensity of urges for sexual pleasure and large-muscle activity increases dramatically with puberty. Anna Freud (1969) described how some adolescents become so frightened by the strength of these impulses, that they may give up pleasures in order to assert mastery over them. Equally important is the recognition that these bodily changes offer the freedom of transforming what was once pure fantasy into potential reality (Laufer and Laufer 1984). Adolescents now have the physical capacity to become parents, and, although it may be difficult for therapists to appreciate, they take great pride in this capacity.

Adolescents also have the newly developed physical capacity to defend themselves against adults or to escape from adults. Whether these new capacities are actually put into use does not obviate the fact that they profoundly affect the new perceptions of the self.

In dealing with these issues it is particularly important for therapists to be aware of their own feelings and attitudes. Adolescent values in regard to sexual behavior may vary substantially from those with which therapists themselves grew up and feel comfortable. Openly or tacitly directing patients to follow certain codes of sexual or ethical behavior—codes that may, in fact, be laden with personal biases—may be a disservice to the patient. This is not to say that discussions about realistic concerns such as pregnancy and sexually transmitted disease should be avoided. But rather, that therapists' personal values in these matters should not be integrated into the therapeutic process. The challenge for therapists is to understand the meaning that these adolescent behaviors and activities have to the youngsters themselves.

Cognitive change.   Adolescence also effects changes in cognitive capacities. Adolescents are often faced with a normative developmental challenge of reorganizing their worldview (Kohlberg and Gilligan 1971). While young children generally want to receive adult approval by being good, and hence following established rules, adolescents may feel compelled to act in accord with their own principles, which sometimes conflict with community rules. This shift in cognitive organization can be highly stressful, demanding the therapist's sympathetic appreciation as well as the recognition that this shift does not ipso facto indicate psychopathology.

Along with this new cognitive capacity come new and more sophisticated modes of defense. For example, upon being told of his obvious sexual conflicts, a teenage boy correctly asserted that the therapist's theoretical orientation made sex a topic of great importance. He then cited conceptual inconsistencies in Freudian thought and offered a reasonable explanation of his problem. The challenge before the therapist was to recognize and acknowledge the patient's intellectual development and, at the same time, help him understand why he was using this development to his own detriment.

In another instance analysis was recommended to a depressed adolescent boy. While he consciously wanted to be in analysis, at some level he was nevertheless ambivalent. In not telling his father of his suffering, and not telling the therapist of his reluctance to discuss this with his father, he was thereby unconsciously arranging an argument between his father and the therapist. Arguing with his father, which was, in fact, playing the assigned role in the boy's externalization defense, got the therapist nowhere. Only when the therapist showed the boy how and why he had arranged the conflict could the difficulty be resolved.

In order to correctly assess similar situations, therapists need to be aware of the fact that adolescents are generally quite interested in the external world and often engaged in some kind of action. They are also typically critical of others. So, while these factors may indicate an attempt to divert attention away from the adolescent's own activities or feelings, they may also be part of normative adolescent style.

Along with cognitive shifting comes a changed sense of self and a search for identity. The central focus of life changes from a present orientation to concern about the future (Galatzer-Levy and Cohler 1990). Adolescents now view themselves as emerging adults—as in the process of becoming, rather than currently being. This transition is only satisfactorily achieved when adolescents feel that they can be themselves.

Although many adolescents achieve this end without passing through the intense and visible identity crises described by Erikson (1968), the theme may play an important role in the treatment process. Patients, especially older adolescents, often use issues of identity and disagreement with the therapist to divert attention away from more pressing therapeutic concerns.

Shifting interdependency.   Although it is agreed that shifts in interdependency occur during adolescence, descriptions of the meaning of these shifts and of the dynamics of the shifting differ substantially. Blos (1967), extending the work of Margaret Mahler (Mahler et al. 1975), describes adolescence as a second separation-individuation. He maintains that adolescents are in a process of becoming more themselves and often struggle mightily with their parents, whom they accuse of interfering with this process. Masterson (1972) and Blos (1983) have written on therapeutic interventions based on this view.

Rather than being a process of becoming independent of other people, development entails shifting patterns of interdependence. Studies of normal young adults and adolescents demonstrate how these individuals become part of the family and community, not separated from them (Cohler and Grunbaum 1981; Offer and Sabshin 1984). Although it has become a norm for middle-class Americans to be very much independent of their parents, there is little empirical indication that this constitutes a model for psychological health. Of course, this is not to say that adolescents do not experience difficulties and vicissitudes with normal interdependence. Separation may not be the major theme for the development of the self as Mahler and Blos contend.

One possible exception to this situation is the case of adolescents who come from severely disturbed families. Unlike most youngsters, they must sometimes become wholly independent from their families if they are to achieve any degree of psychological growth.

Working Alliances

Alliance With Patients

The working alliance with adolescents is based on the same fundamental principle as alliances with other patients. That is, the extent to which patients and therapists collaborate in reaching shared goals profoundly affects outcome. A clear-cut failure to address and resolve this issue may sometimes lead to interrupted treatments. In cases where adolescents actually enact a charade of self-exploration in order to be with the therapist or to serve as the "admission price" to therapy, the psychotherapeutic process can go on indefinitely without useful results. Such manipulation may be only one of several possible causes for the working alliance disappearing. For therapy to lead to the patient's resumption of growth, therapists must understand these causes and overcome any impediments to collaboration.

To a great extent therapists must allow adolescents to define their needs. Often therapists have an implicit agenda in mind as they work with patients and misinterpret their patients' failure to follow that agenda as a problem that needs to be surmounted. Absence from therapy, failure to talk, or talking about seemingly unimportant matters can be understood as ways of avoiding important issues. While in many instances this may be true, these occurrences may also represent valuable developmental activities of which the therapist is not yet aware.

This is exemplified in the case of a high school student who spent much of his time in treatment discussing current movies. His descriptions were vivid and insightful, and a pleasure to listen to. The treatment went well, but periodic movie reports continued throughout the treatment period. Near the end of treatment, when the boy was in the midst of working on issues that deeply concerned him, he began a session by giving a lengthy report on a film. When the therapist suggested to the boy that this was a way to avoid talking more directly about other matters, the boy was quite surprised. After all, he had been doing this for several months, and the therapist had enjoyed listening. The therapist finally asked directly, "Why do you always talk about movies?" The boy replied, "Because you are the only one who will listen." The boy's family was highly critical of him, and much of his low self-esteem arose from the fact that they could not enjoy his talents. When he revealed his artistic and critical sensibility in therapy sessions, the therapist provided a much-needed receptive audience for this vital and underappreciated aspect of his self.

Commonly, adolescents miss many appointments. The assumption that they are not engaged in treatment when this happens is often mistaken. During her high school years a flighty teenage girl arrived at least 15 minutes late for only the third appointment that she had kept. Despite the fact that the sessions were usually passed in discussions of lipstick and nail polish colors, the therapist maintained a position of interest and respect. Sensing that there was more to the girl than the flibbertigibbet she presented, the therapist offered interpretations of her motives and anxieties. As the patient neared the end of high school, her attendance became even more erratic. Several years later, however, while engaged in a rigorous academic program, she wrote to the therapist telling him how vitally important it had been to her that he had remained available and had taken her seriously, even though she had "blown off" the therapy.

Alliance With Parents

Although adolescents frequently complain about their parents and talk of their independence from them, they nevertheless maintain an incredible degree of loyalty toward them. Therapists should be aware of this emotion. In many ways, parents remain the center of the world—the surest source of support and solace for adolescents.

Successful treatment thus requires that therapists maintain good working alliances with parents, and most parents who are approached in a spirit of reason and commitment to the well-being of their child are supportive of treatment. Therapists cannot, however, just assume that parents understand either their adolescent's psychology or the therapeutic process. They should, in fact, begin with the assumption that parents know very little about these matters, and proceed to spell out exactly what they are doing and why.

Being told that one's child is in serious psychological difficulty is painful and frightening for parents. When they are concerned about poignant and urgent questions pertaining to what they have done wrong or what their child's future is, they must be allowed adequate time to work through these issues with the therapist. Their doubts and questions and their need to get to know the therapist indicate concern; these responses should not be misconstrued as resistance. Therapists' anxieties about getting to work on the "real" problems, and their failure to spend the time necessary to develop an adequate alliance with parents, commonly result in the interruption or sabotaging of treatment. This can happen even when parents themselves are not paying for treatment, for they may still feel threatened or unsafe.

A less abrupt but equally significant course of action may also be taken by parents who feel that therapists are unresponsive to their needs. They may unconsciously feel forced to communicate by interfering with the therapeutic approach. They may fail to pay bills in a timely fashion or introduce scheduling constraints that make therapy impossible. These problems are generally not "administrative problems." Rather, they are important indications that more flexible and effective channels of communication need to be developed. To ignore them is to put therapy in peril.

A difficult set of problems may arise in alliances with parents who are divorced. Often issues of responsibility for payment become the manifest way of trying to attribute blame for the child's psychopathology. Because children of divorce almost always remain loyal to both parents, manifest or latent conflicts add to the difficulties they are experiencing. Every effort should therefore be made to establish an alliance with both parents—even when one seems entirely uninvolved in the treatment.

When there is a real disparity between the goals of parent and child and the child begins to successfully address important issues, the parent may interrupt treatment. Recognizing and addressing such situations can sometimes lead to their management and sometimes result in retreating from these situations in order to avoid introducing yet more grief into the patient's life. To illustrate, a 16-year-old girl lived with her father, who was embittered at his ex-wife. He viewed his ex-wife as promiscuous, as a spendthrift, and as a drug abuser, and feared that his daughter would grow up like her. After the divorce the girl refused to visit the mother, who, in any case, seemed uninterested in her. As treatment progressed it emerged that the girl's incompletely consolidated identification with her mother represented a vital aspect of her personality. Her refusal to see her mother grew out of her own rage at her mother, as well as compliance with her father's wishes. As a result of treatment she decided to reestablish contact, and did so, much to her pleasure and psychological benefit. The father, however, became furious. He felt betrayed and consequently forced the interruption of therapy.

Cases such as this one are instances in which family treatment or other interventions with the family are essential if the adolescent is to develop and change. Because many adolescents use externalization to transform internal difficulties into family problems, it is often difficult to determine when resistance to change has its origin primarily within an adolescent and when the family environment is that which precludes change. Careful consideration should be given to both possibilities.

Confidentiality

Aware of the fact that therapists have special knowledge of their adolescent, parents commonly seek their guidance in managing the child. This of course puts therapists in a difficult position, for they must protect the privacy of their patients' communications. In the long run their demonstrated understanding of why parents need special information in order to make decisions is more valuable than their actually providing parents with information.

Because this situation is unlike all other situations in which parents are entitled to know about their child, clear explanations for the arrangement should be given. Patients need to be aware of the fact that if their parents are to continue supporting therapy, they must be informed of the general progress being made. Patients should also know that should they act in dangerous ways, special interventions may be required. Similarly, parents must be made to realize that secret communications with therapists lead to an adolescent's expanded fantasies, and that although the patient's communications to the therapists are confidential, the parents' communications may well be discussed with the child. Laying out these rules of confidentiality early in the treatment generally avoids later difficulty in this area.

Transference

The General Concept

In this chapter the term "transference" is used to refer to the patient's important psychological positions with regard to the therapist. As with other perceptions, these positions are the result of an active process—the patient's construction of the world based on needs and wishes as well as selected incoming stimuli. Although transferences need not involve repetitions of past experience, they often do.

While transferences are generally shifting configurations, central themes that may constitute a relatively complete and important structure in the patient's life often emerge. The degree of clarity attained concerning transferences largely depends on the therapeutic stance.

The major function of the psychoanalytic model is to permit the unclouded emergence of transferences, their elucidation, and their interpretation. When analysts see patients frequently and over an extended period of time, they systematically attempt to remove the impediments to their patients' speaking freely. Transferences thus surface with clarity and can be explored to a degree to which they seldom can in other types of approaches.

Transference Phenomena in Adolescents

While many transference configurations occur during adolescence, certain configurations are seen more commonly. These include hostility to all "grown-ups," idealization, mirroring transference, issues about being one's own person, and oedipal transference. One major problem that arises is a tendency on the part of therapists to enact a complementary role to transferences rather than to use them to enlarge the joint understanding and mastery of the adolescent's psychological world. This tendency is easily understandable, for it is natural for adults to want to meet the psychological needs of adolescents and to fall into the trap of believing that they are uniquely able to fulfill the adolescents' psychological requirements.

Aichhorn (1925) understood pervasive negativity toward all adults as reflecting disappointed idealization. His approach to these transferences, which imperil the formation of any alliance, was to manipulate the situation so that he became the object of intense idealization. For example, in his work with a delinquent youngster he might beat him at billiards or he might demonstrate how much more clever he was than the boy at planning a robbery. A simpler, less complicated approach is to maintain a stance of interest in the patient and in the reason for his or her current feelings. This in itself is likely to be a surprise to youngsters accustomed to provoking angry responses from adults.

Idealizing transferences may be either ordinary transient adolescent idealization or transferences emerging from archaic needs for an idealizable figure (the latter being characteristic of disorders of the self) (Kohut and Wolf 1978). Although similar in many ways, these transferences differ both in their clinical manifestations and in their implications for the patient's psychological structure.

Interferences with ordinary adolescent idealizations usually 1) are the result of actual maturation (i.e., the patient begins to see the therapist more realistically), or 2) occur when therapists behave in such a way that patients lose some degree of respect for them. Such instances usually result in disappointment or minor functional disturbances in which the patient's core self is not threatened. Because this form of idealization is a prominent feature of ordinary adolescent development, it is not surprising that it appears in treatment.

In contrast, when an idealization that reflects early developmental needs is interrupted, the patient feels fragmented and depleted of energy and undertakes some impulsive compensatory action. Such interruptions often result from breaks in the therapeutic alliance or failures on the part of therapists that, to the external observer, may be relatively minor.

A second type of transference involves "mirroring," or a sense of being vigorous, good, and cohesive because of the environment's appreciation or because one shares a position in the world with another—a "twinship." As with idealizing transferences, mirroring transferences may reflect either early deficits in development or current, age-appropriate developmental needs. And as with idealization, the differentiation is made on the basis of the patient's degree of disturbance in response to interferences with the mirroring transference (Kohut 1971).

Many adolescents are preoccupied with being their own person and fear that therapists will interfere. This sometimes represents a reaction against fears of being psychologically enslaved, but more often reflects the underlying feeling that to be one's own person one must be independent of others. Adolescents may believe that therapists are trying to influence them for their own purposes, and hence feel that they cannot be themselves. Such ideas can arise from the experience of having had to fulfill the psychological goals and needs of others. Therapists' responses to such transferences should thus be based on an understanding of their meaning, and therapists should attempt to assist patients in distinguishing internal wishes and fears from external realities. Assertions by therapists that they are not really as they are seen are of little value.

Another possible transference is the repetition in therapy of the oedipal situation. Even for the vast majority of youngsters who certainly do not directly enact oedipal longings, the combination of intensified drive and the physical possibility of enacting this wish is a severe strain. The intensity of the wishes and fears directed toward therapists often terrifies youngsters.

A frequent problem is the therapist's failure to understand the difficulty of the situation even for seemingly sophisticated adolescents. Although some adolescents may have considerable sexual experience and talk freely about erotic matters, they may still feel frightened and humiliated about their sexual feelings toward the therapist. In essence, much of the generational separation is a reinstatement of the incest taboo in slightly modified form, and therapists who fail to appreciate the intensity of this taboo are likely to traumatize or at least needlessly frighten their patients.

Countertransference

Countertransference, or the therapist's transference to the patient, is an inevitable aspect of the therapeutic encounter. As with other transferences, it arises as a result of both the stimulating aspects of the environment (i.e., the patient) and the therapist's unconscious wishes and needs.

Countertransferences can be useful to treatment when they are systematically explored as a tool for understanding patients by way of analysts' unconscious responses to them (Racker 1968). They can interfere with the treatment when they lead therapists to distort their basic therapeutic stance in response to their feelings toward patients.

With therapists' knowledge and mastery of their own transferences comes the increased likelihood that they will be able to use the countertransference as a source of useful therapeutic information. However, adolescents' use of externalization and the intensities of their transferences often make concomitant countertransference responses more intense and more problematic than those with other age groups.

Countertransferences to adolescents are frequently determined by the developmental stage of therapists themselves. Many young therapists who are just starting out have not yet settled into adulthood and still view the "adult" generation as alien. Difficulties may then arise as a result of counteridentification with patients—the therapists' feelings that they themselves are adolescents. Such a feeling is a double-edged sword, for on the one hand, it can motivate therapists to intense interest in matters in which other adults might have little psychological investment. On the other hand, this feeling can also lead to a lack of objectivity in assessing the adolescent's worldview.

Problems also arise when a patient experiences a therapist as an adult when, in fact, the therapist wants and expects to be experienced as a peer. In such instances, much valuable time can be wasted as the therapist tries to convince the patient that he or she shares a similar outlook on the world.

As therapists age and often become parents themselves, they are more likely to identify with parents' positions and feelings and to notice parental elements in their transferences. Insofar as their own identification with this role interferes with understanding the world through the adolescent's eyes, it interferes with therapy. Moreover, the common illusion that the therapist can provide parental functions that the child is not currently receiving or did not receive is also likely to lead to complications in treatment.

Realistic concerns in the area of sex, drugs, and violence are often admixed with moral positions, and the latter are then equated with realistic issues. For example, a prominent psychiatrist of conservative moral, political, and religious conviction appeared on television advocating abstinence as the surest prevention of AIDS, and described the value of abstinence in adolescents' psychological development. He apparently believed that the basis of this view lay not in his moral system, but rather in his knowledge of the epidemiology of AIDS and the nature of normal adolescent development.

In a subtler instance, an adolescent boy was in treatment with a psychiatrist who had formerly been active in the civil rights movement. The boy repeatedly talked with contempt about various racial groups. It was clear that these groups represented unacceptable elements of himself that were evidenced in other ways also discussed. But the patient, and later the therapist, became aware that the therapist was consistently much more active in interpreting this particular displacement than others. Under the guise of interpretation, the therapist was engaging in a kind of moral education that interfered with listening to and understanding the patient.

The physical vigor, beauty, and limitless range of opportunities open to adolescents commonly elicit the envy of therapists. Likewise, these youngsters' competitiveness and demands to be admired for supposed accomplishments often precipitate feelings of contempt. As with moral positions, these feelings in therapists often manifest as "educational" positions. A youngster beaming with pride brought an "A" term paper for the therapist to read and received a critique as though she were writing for a scholarly journal. The therapist believed that he was contributing to the patient's intellectual development.

While the adolescent's tendency to manage internal distress by creating external situations often exerts intense pressure on the therapist to play an assigned role, this counterresponse is an essential aspect of the deep alliance between therapist and patient. The previously described case in which an adolescent boy's conflict about whether to enter analysis was played out as an argument between the boy's father and the therapist required considerable work on the part of the therapist, including consultation with a colleague, before he understood what was occurring and the role he was playing. Counterresponses, however, can provide rich insight into the psychology of patients and their interpersonal styles.

Termination of Therapy

For the therapist, ending work with an adolescent who has come to be valued and appreciated can be a sad experience. For the patient, termination of treatment involves a conscious and unconscious review and reworking of the entire therapeutic process. Ultimately, it involves mourning the loss of both the treatment and the therapist. This experience is generally painful, necessitating close collaboration so as to minimize the intensity and emotional impact. The youngster's state of well-being, the therapist's pride in the work accomplished, and the socially syntonic optimism of youth can all be used to obscure the mourning.

Structuring the period of termination by the therapist so that the experience of loss is nontraumatic allows adolescents to sort and shift those parts of the experience that will be internalized as part of their own psyche and those that will not. Under pressure of time, they will hopefully come to explore issues that they realize cannot be postponed forever.

Perfectionistic ideas about what should be accomplished in psychotherapy often lead therapists and patients to believe that seeking further treatment is an indication of failure in the first therapy. This is quite incorrect. To the contrary, patients who discover the benefits of treatment at one point in their lives are likely to use it again when it is appropriate. When patients seek further psychotherapy, it usually indicates that they have found their previous experiences useful.

Conclusions

The dynamic nature of adolescence manifests in an ongoing series of challenges to therapists. In addition to having general psychotherapeutic expertise, therapists must also have a thorough understanding of the special dimensions of adolescent behavior and their possible impact on treatment. They must be aware of the physical and cognitive changes that adolescents experience, as well as the shifting patterns of interdependency. They must grasp the complexities of their working alliances and of transference phenomena, and realize the roles that these respectively play in the therapeutic outcome. Finally, therapists must know how to structure the period of termination so as to lessen the feeling of loss.

Within this framework, the key factor is understanding—not manipulating, not controlling, and not educating. And only through this understanding can therapists lead their adolescent patients toward the resumption of growth and the realization of their patients' own inner goals.

References

Aichhorn A: Wayward Youth. London, Imago, 1925
Blos P: The second individuation process of adolescence. Psychoanal Study Child 22:162–186, 1967

Blos P: The contribution of psychoanalysis to the psychotherapy of adolescents. Psychoanal Study Child 38:577–600, 1983

Cohler B., Grunbaum H: Mothers, Grandmothers, and Daughters. New York, John Wiley, 1981

Erikson E: Identity, Youth, and Crisis. New York, WW Norton, 1968

Freud A: Adolescence (1958), in Research at the Hampstead Child-Therapy Clinic and Other Papers (1956–1965). The Writings of Anna Freud, Vol 5. New York, International Universities Press, 1969, pp 136–166

Galatzer-Levy R: On working through: a model from artificial intelligence. J Am Psychoanal Assoc 26:125–150, 1988

Galatzer-Levy R, Cohler B: The Essential Other. New York, Basic Books, 1990

Kohlberg L, Gilligan C: The adolescent as a philosopher: the discovery of the self in the post-conventional world. Daedalus 100:1051–1086, 1971

Kohut H: The Analysis of the Self: A Systematic Approach to the Psychoanalytic Treatment of Narcissistic Personality Disorders. New York, International Universities Press, 1971

Kohut H, Wolf E: Disorders of the self and their treatment: an outline. Int J Psychoanal 59:413–425, 1978

Laufer M, Laufer M: Adolescence and Developmental Breakdown. New Haven, CT, Yale University Press, 1984

Mahler M, Pine F, Bergman A: The Psychological Birth of the Human Infant. New York, Basic Books, 1975

Masterson J: Treatment of the Borderline Adolescent: A Developmental Approach. New York, Wiley-Interscience, 1972

Offer D, Sabshin M: Adolescence: empirical perspectives, in Normality and the Life Cycle. Edited by Offer D, Sabshin M. New York, Basic Books, 1984, pp 76–107

Racker H: Transference and Counter-Transference. New York, International Universities Press, 1968

Weiss S: Reflections on the psychoanalytic process, with special emphasis on child analysis and self analysis. Annual for Psychoanalysis 9:43–56, 1981

Group Psychotherapy of Adolescents

SAUL SCHEIDLINGER, Ph.D.
SETH ARONSON, Psy.D.

Chapter 6

Group Psychotherapy of Adolescents

*T*he very thought of adolescence conjures up in one's mind the notion of group life. Adolescents indisputably spend more of their waking hours in groups than in any other context. The typical American high school comprises at least six different peer-group structures ranging in hierarchical order from the college-bound "brains" or "jocks," at the top, to the secretly admired yet feared, tough "greasers," at the bottom. (The small number of unaffiliated youths, often termed "duds," are in fact the most likely candidates for some kind of mental health intervention.)

The adolescent peer group serves a crucial role in the promotion of self-esteem and of social and moral maturation, and, above all, in the emancipation from the family. The peer group is a refuge—there is safety in numbers. It is thus reassuring for a teenager to note that others are also awkward, have acne, and are mixed up about bodily changes and about sexuality.

Sullivan (1953) spoke of preadolescent "chums" as precursors to intimate relationships. Blos (1979) noted that the adolescent group, with its defensive inclination to split the adult world into good and bad, may afford teenagers the opportunity to unify the idealized and depreciated parental images. This natural propensity for group affiliation together with a hesitancy to rely on adults makes the group therapy approach a sensible and practical treatment of choice for this age group.

Group Helping Modalities for Adolescents

Group work with adolescents occurs in many different contexts. Scheidlinger (1985) described four distinct, yet related categories of "group helping" modalities for teenagers. The first of these categories refers to *group psychotherapy proper.* The second category was termed *therapeutic groups*; the third, *human development and training groups*; and the last category, *self-help and mutual-help groups.*

It is useful to view these four categories of group modalities as more or less planned efforts to promote behavioral change in individual adolescents. Although basically different, they share selected motivational factors and techniques. In this connection the following four interrelated variables are worthy of special consideration:

1. The *leader–change agent variable*, which includes the latter's training, theoretical persuasion, and objectives for the group.
2. The *client variable*, which refers to such characteristics as each given youth's sex, age, sociocultural background, and expectations about the group undertaking.
3. The *methodology variable*, which entails the service provider's preference for specific techniques within the confines of his or her broader assumptions regarding the promotion of desired behavior change in the participants.
4. The *process variable*, which reflects the totality of what the service provider believes to be happening in the group experience.

A brief overview of the nature of each of the earlier noted four categories of group helping modalities for adolescents is given below.

Category I.   Group psychotherapy is a specific clinical modality lodged in the broader field of the psychotherapies. A trained mental health professional uses the emotional interaction among participants in a small, carefully balanced group to effect amelioration of personality difficulties in individuals specifically selected for this purpose. Each group member has a diagnosed problem and views the group experience as a means of modifying his or her psychological functioning.

Category II.   "Therapeutic" groups addressed to designated adolescent patients in mental health settings include all the group approaches (other than group psychotherapy) that are used by human services personnel in inpatient or outpatient facilities. In inpatient settings examples would be therapeutic community, occupational therapy, and art or dance therapy, as well as special education groups. In residential schools for delinquent or neglected youths, milieu or behavior modification groups, as well as "rap" sessions, are typical. Similar approaches are utilized in the many "alternative" high schools and day treatment programs for teenagers. In outpatient settings there can be short-term waiting list or diagnostic groups, including discussion groups for adolescents with chronic medical diseases such as diabetes or multiple sclerosis.

Category III. Human development and training groups belong more to the realm of affective and cognitive education than to therapeutics. They range, on the one hand, from public consciousness-raising and sensitivity-training groups, to, on the other hand, the variously-termed human relations or group counseling endeavors employed in high schools. The mushrooming school-based educational groupings aimed at preventing substance abuse, unplanned pregnancies, venereal diseases, and especially AIDS, would belong here as well.

Category IV. Self-help and mutual-help groups generally represent voluntary group structures for mutual aid and for the accomplishment of a general purpose. This model has been specifically applied to adolescents in the field of substance abuse wherein the Synanon or Alcoholics Anonymous approach is used with youths in residential or community programs.

Even though it is often difficult to chart exact boundaries among the four broad categories of group helping modalities for adolescents delineated above, such an attempt is nevertheless preferable to the confusion one finds in the literature and in practice.

Whom to Include in a Therapy Group and Why

Slavson (1950) has emphasized the importance of selecting group members carefully in order to achieve a group balance. Level of psychosexual development should be noted, and such variables as sex, age, socioeconomic and educational background, and specific pathologies should also be considered. Thus, not only is it necessary to ask if the patient is likely to benefit from group therapy, but a second question is relevant as well: is this particular group suitable for this patient?

While, broadly speaking, there is some kind of group for every disturbed adolescent (i.e., the earlier-noted "therapeutic" groups), nondirective outpatient therapy groups are unsuitable for youths with active psychoses, for those in crisis, or for those with severe sexual or addictive disorders. In addition, the frequently employed model of psychodynamically geared, permissive talking groups is counterindicated for adolescents who are acutely vulnerable to emotional disclosures, to confrontation, and to contagious behavior. Such youths, including overly impulsive ones, function best in homogeneous, structured groups with explicit limits, rules, and expectations. Gardner (1988) found it useful to include a selected few antisocial patients in his heterogeneous groups, because being in a minority helped these antisocial individuals to recognize the narrowness of their repertoire.

In some instances, where a prospective group member's "fit" is difficult to predict, an invitation to visit an ongoing group for a trial period is advisable. The following case study illustrates this point:

> Anthony, a 15-year-old Italian boy, came to this multiethnic group as a "visitor." The therapist was not sure how this shy and anxious youngster would fare in a group that contained some severely hyperactive and impulsive boys. As it turned out, Anthony attached himself from the start to a younger Hispanic boy whom he had known from summer day camp. In addition, Anthony's skill in ping-pong made him a sought-out partner in games. He soon became an accepted member of the group and appeared to enjoy it to the point where he did not miss a single session. When spring came, with the help of his renewed confidence and burgeoning social skills, Anthony tried out for the school baseball team and was selected pitcher. With daily team practice after school, the boy chose reluctantly to terminate from the group. The therapist viewed this as a desirable development.

Group therapy is generally considered to be the treatment of choice for most adolescents. It has been found to be especially effective with youngsters who are deficient in social skills, with those suffering from low self-esteem, or with those having particular difficulties in trusting adult authority figures.

Individual preparatory sessions with all candidates for group therapy are desirable practice. These sessions are useful for purposes of screening, and for those patients deemed acceptable, they can also be used as a means to establish a therapeutic alliance in the less threatening one-to-one setting. In addition, the latter offers an opportunity to deal with the patient's understandable concerns and questions about the projected group experience.

Many therapists prefer to see their adolescent patients concurrently in both individual and group treatment. The group modality is usually added after a period of individual contacts. In such "combined" therapy, the dyadic sessions then serve to complement the intense input from the group experience, allowing for the slower process of "working through" to occur (Scheidlinger 1982).

Groups for Younger and for Older Adolescents

Mental health professionals are quite familiar with the difficulty of establishing a therapeutic relationship with early adolescents (ages 13–15) because of their almost uncontrollable restlessness and need to defend their beginning autonomy against adults. Massive denial, externalization, concrete thinking, and orientation to the present all work against attempts to promote meaningful communications leading to self-awareness. A group setting that allows for free motility and that combines activities, games, and snacks with periods of discussion has been found most appropriate for this population. Even in a group, however, younger adolescents are likely to be self-conscious. There is much squirming, kidding around, and whispering to pals. Warm feelings addressed to the adult can be supplanted by anger within a short time span. In contrast to the usually coeducational *talking* groups most suited to the needs of older adolescents, mixing of the sexes in group work with younger adolescents leads usually to countertherapeutic anxiety levels.

The following account drawn from an early session of an early adolescent boys' group conveys the tone of the treatment process:

The emotions liberated by the advent of a new member (who was luckily strong enough to hold his attackers at bay) signaled the end of the group's relatively calm honeymoon period. With the sudden emergence of distinct, troubled individuals, propelled by inner anxieties, the prevailing nonverbal message now seemed to be: "Where do I fit in this group?" Pulled in many directions by the acter-outers, the therapist had to limit behavior, explain, support, and occasionally exclude individuals temporarily from the room for them to calm down and get a hold of themselves.

Compare this account with a glimpse at an early session of a coeducational group of 17-year-old girls and boys, as chronicled by the presiding therapist:

As was true last week, our circle held three girls to my left and the four boys to my right. After they had helped themselves to the Cokes and to the chips there was some separate whispering and giggling among the girls and among the boys. Then followed an awkward silence with expectant glances directed at me. When no one responded to my invitation to remind the group about last week's discussion, I said: "You know last time there was the feeling expressed that being a teenager today is harder than before. You mentioned money, drugs, and you began to touch on dealing with parents. What about that?" Jane: "I am pissed at my mother. We had a still bigger hassle last night. Now, I'm going out with a friend, not even a boyfriend—she's just a girl I'm hanging out with. My mother wants to meet this friend and yells that I better be back by 10:00." Phyllis: "When my mother starts giving me this kind of shit, I don't listen to her; I walk out, I don't care." Karen: "Some of these restrictions can be quite outrageous. Like they want you home for dinner at 6:00, no matter what happens, no matter where you are. Like you have to take a plane home and be there for dinner. That's so stupid!" I observed that all the boys had so far stayed silent. John smiled broadly and said: "Cause that's the way it has to be for girls. They can get in trouble—like some guys messing around with them. . . . It's the same with my mother and my sister."

In view of the particular difficulty of early adolescents in addressing themselves to anything even approaching self-awareness, careful timing of verbal interventions is necessary, as the following illustrates:

In one group of early-adolescent boys, the boys were very reluctant to discuss controlling their anger. The leaders felt it was wise to allow the group time to feel comfortable discussing the issue. After several months, the boys requested a specific craft project—they wanted to make volcanoes from clay, baking soda, and vinegar. Upon making the volcanoes they began to talk freely about their problems of anger "erupting," and a meaningful discussion ensued with references to their discipline problems at school.

Common Themes in Adolescent Group Psychotherapy

Many authors have concerned themselves with the themes of adolescence. Blos (1962, 1979), A. Freud (1958), and Adelson and Doehrman (1980) described the psychoanalytic motifs of this period: a reactivation of oedipal and preoedipal conflicts as well as those of separation-individuation. Variations and echoes of these themes occur in groups. Of special note here are the defenses often used by adolescents (e.g., oral greediness, anal humor, pseudomaturity), all reflecting inner and outer conflicts.

Although these themes may be consistent for teenagers of all ages, some concerns come to the fore while others recede during different developmental phases. For example, the time variations in the physiological maturing of girls and boys may give rise to certain unique psychosocial issues in an early adolescent group (i.e., the more mature girls complaining about the boys' relative immaturity).

As might be expected, relationships to parents and to other authority figures constitute a pervasive theme in all adolescent groups. In this connection there is an acute awareness of how adults regard them, and the adolescents are sensitive to any sign of suspicion or distrust directed toward them. Such signals only serve to fuel the adolescents' self-doubt and arouse anxiety regarding their sense of competency.

Management of sexual impulses coupled with questions about the capacity for intimacy and solidification of sexual identity is in the foreground. Concerns regarding homosexuality, masturbation, or simply the need for elementary sex education are ever present, as in the following case:

> In an early-adolescent boys' group, many of the youths had questions regarding sex. However, the topic was too sensitive and emotionally laden, leading repeatedly to anxious giggling and teasing. After several months some boys responded to the leader's offer to bring in illustrated materials on sex education. Despite their veneer of being "street-wise smart," the boys showed astonishingly little knowledge of elementary facts such as how a baby is conceived and born.

In due time the group eventually allows adolescents to examine the nature of their relationships and the consequences of sexual activities. Above all, the honest interchanges lead the boys and girls to begin to regard each other as fellow human beings and not simply as objects for gratification.

Such discussions may, in turn, lead to themes of family, of adult relationships, and of the successes and pitfalls of marriage. Questions around single-parent families, conflicted marital relationships that the adolescents may experience first-hand, and coping with parents' boyfriends or girlfriends also arise.

MacLennan and Felsenfeld (1968) as well as Rachman (1972) elaborated on the ways group therapy helps to solidify adolescents' sense of identity. Such subjects as today's "me" generation versus altruism (i.e., making money or helping others) and society's double message of fostering dependency yet demanding adult demeanor are frequently talked about in groups for older adolescents.

With a degree of trust and cohesion established, the inevitable alliances and conflicts in the group itself can become the subject of sincere scrutiny. A nondefensive posture is critical; here, the members need to recognize that differences arise and can be worked out and negotiated with appropriate concern and regard for all. The group therapist's willingness to also look at and discuss his or her own behavior serves as a potent model in this connection. In all groups, therapeutic efforts must be directed at getting individuals to talk out rather than act upon feelings. This is no small order for a population in which denial, externalization, grandiosity, and problems in delaying gratification are so common.

The above kinds of anxiety-laden themes cannot be maintained in the group for long. Accordingly, alternating periods of emotionally charged *work* and of *rest* through various diversionary tactics such as uncomfortable silences, light banter, or intellectualizing, are commonplace. The following example from a coeducational group of 16- and 17-year-olds portrays this process, including the appropriate therapist interventions:

> Dorothy began the session saying tearfully: "My old man came home last night and found my mother drunk again. They were screaming at each other and I didn't sleep a wink." The other group members appeared to pay no attention to Dorothy, as they kidded around, teasing each other. Jeremy and David even began blowing the paper from their drinking straws at the girls. The therapist changed the course of the session: "I'm puzzled by the goings on here and especially with your failing to attend to what Dorothy is saying. Could it be that it is too painful to be reminded of the disappointing behavior of your parents?"

The youths froze in silence. After some discomforted glances away from the adult, they began, one by one, to tell their own stories. A boy exclaimed, "You think you got it bad. My father gambled away all the money we had on the stock market and lost his job to boot." Another girl revealed that her father was having an affair with his secretary: "Can you imagine the shame! And this is the same man who lectured me only last week about my dating two guys on the same Saturday." "You see, Dorothy, you are not alone," the therapist said. Following some such further exchanges about parental "misbehavior," another silence settled. With it went again an eyeing of fingers, of the table, or of the floor—anything to avoid looking at the adult. This time, instead of confronting the youths again with their resistance to work further on these issues, the therapist suggested: "It seems to me that the group has reached a point of needing a rest from spilling so much heavy stuff all at once. You might want to pick up from here next week."

In succeeding sessions, the supportive group guided by the therapist attempts to help its members focus in greater detail on such serious problems at home or on relationships with their contemporaries. Realistic assessments of each situation should lead to thoughtful decisions instead of to acting on impulse.

Phases of Group Development and Appropriate Therapist Techniques

Psychotherapy groups move through identifiable developmental phases. In the early stages, termed "pre-affiliation" and "power and control" (Garland et al. 1973), the members first try to get acquainted while competing with simultaneous wishes to maintain a protective distance. The question of who is to be trusted is paramount. "What will the leader and the others think of me?" "Will I be exposed or turned away?" These are just a few of the characteristic concerns.

In this initial period of generalized anxiety and of testing, the therapist, being the central person in the group, needs to be clear about how much and what kind of behavior will be tolerated. The "power and control" phase is bound to be especially trying for the adult, since it is characterized by much contagious rebelliousness and struggles for status with fluctuating role assignments (i.e., scapegoat, clown, peacemaker). While projecting himself or herself as an accepting, caring yet firm person, the therapist conveys his or her understanding of the insecurity inherent in such a new experience. The therapist must demonstrate the ability to control harmful behavior, coupled with a belief that, once coalesced, the group will move to its appointed task: to share problems and feelings and to work on these. This will require a climate of trust wherein the members will feel free to express any ideas or feelings without fear of censure.

A number of authors have written about the varied individual and group defenses that characterize adolescent groups, especially in their early phases. Thus, Redl (1966) denoted such defenses as escape into love, protective provocation, and escape from guilt. MacLennan and Felsenfeld (1968) described various diversionary maneuvers, among them arguing, monopolizing, scapegoating, and silence. Rosenthal (1971) focused on the way individual defensive denial and projection are intertwined with group elements. (The handling of these defensive manifestations will be discussed in a later section of this chapter.)

During a group's middle phase is when truly intensive work can occur. With the major issue of trust resolved, and a therapeutic alliance consolidated, verbal interventions ranging from clarifications through confrontations to interpretations, can be employed in the service of self-awareness and of insight regarding the conscious and unconscious motivational factors that underlie behavior. In their role as "peer therapists," other group members are likely to be especially helpful here in the handling of the typical adolescent denials and projections, and in the testing of reality. For one's peers are invariably perceived as less suspect and threatening than even the most benign adult authority figure of the therapist. The therapist's task during this phase is also to provide a balance between anxiety-laden confrontations and support. He or she needs to promote behavior that will lead to enhanced group cohesion while at the same time focusing on the importance of translating insights into action.

The final phase is that of termination. Whether the group has met for a long term or a short term, such a meaningful interpersonal experience is bound to evoke reactions to the impending separation. As is true in individual treatment, some regressions to earlier behavior may occur. In their wish to avoid experiencing the pain of separation, adolescents often try to downplay the profound feelings inherent in this situation. With patient support and some prodding from the therapist the sense of loss and of mourning is eventually brought to the fore. Not infrequently, together with the poignant "good-byes" goes a dramatic reliving of the group's history, coupled with realistic assessments of each member's "progress" and lack of "progress." Behavioral rehearsals and role playing for what lies ahead in the world outside are helpful here as a way of stressing the positives inherent in independent functioning.

Needless to say, group leaders must also monitor their own feelings toward the termination, for the experience is bound to have had significant meanings for them as well.

Adult and Adolescent Groups: A Comparison

In an article aptly entitled "Parent, Teacher or Analyst: The Adolescent Group Therapist's Trilemma," Phelan (1974) outlined the significant conceptual and technical differences between adult and adolescent psychotherapy groups.

For adolescents flexibility and pragmatism are a must. The all important initial task is that of creating a workable group. In contrast with the nondirective stance appropriate for adult groups, the adolescent group therapist is an outgoing, actively involved, and openly friendly person. Furthermore, instructions, encouragement, and directiveness are expected therapeutic functions. The adult has to serve as a role model through the way he or she handles direct questions as well as the ever-present provocations from the group. Both spontaneous and responsive self-disclosures from the therapist, offered within limits of propriety, are often cited by adolescent patients as having been the decisive factors in the establishment of a trusting therapeutic relationship.

Expensively furnished and carpeted meeting rooms are counterindicated for adolescent groups. Rooms for early adolescents should resemble an arts and crafts workshop with space for active games and a round table for refreshments. Older adolescents are best served in a lounge-type setting with comfortable chairs arranged around, for example, a coffee table.

The first session, following the introductions, should begin with a discussion of the group "contract." The contract includes expectations about attendance, the purpose of the group, and forbidden behaviors such as coming to a session "stoned" or drunk, hurting others, or defacing property. There is an interchange about confidentiality, with the *rule* that session content is not to be shared with anyone outside the group. The therapist's promise of confidentiality includes a proviso that he or she will be bound to disclose information that is threatening to any member's health and safety. In coeducational groups, the undesirability of "dating" among group members is explained.

Typical countertransference reactions in adolescent group therapists differ from those operative in adult group therapy. To begin with, in all work with adolescents, countertransference manifestations are more frequent perhaps because of the larger number of unresolved issues remaining with people from that developmental stage. As with most parents, there can be simply the latent envy of the adolescent's youth, vitality, and physique. Adolescent "crushes" on adults carry a strong emotional charge calling for mature understanding and sensitive handling. Then there are the more complex phenomena discussed by Azima (1972) ranging from over-identification with the youths as victims of unsympathetic adults to perfectionistic expectations (i.e., "my parents were much tougher on me and I did okay"). All countertransference manifestations are handled most easily in the context of supervision or perhaps in discussion with cotherapists or other professional peers.

There is no agreement in the field as to whether the general admonition against cotherapy in group therapy for adults should hold for adolescent groups as well. Our experience is similar to that of Davis and Lohr (1971): cotherapy is preferable in the training of new practitioners and in all group work with severely disturbed and especially with such hard-to-reach youths as delinquent or substance-abusing individuals. Many experienced private practitioners, however, who tend to employ combined individual and group treatment seem to be more comfortable and effective as solo group therapists.

Some Problem Group Behaviors and Difficult Members

Clinicians working with adolescents are likely to encounter many moments when they are openly challenged and even provoked. For example, a court-referred youth said to the therapist: "I'm bored in here and wish you'd do more to make this a better group." Instead of turning this issue to the group (i.e., "What do the others think?") and thus inviting a possible collusion, it might be best to tackle such challenges head on. A response such as "Tell me more about what you would like from me," or "What would you like me to do differently?" should convey the adult's desired forthright and nondefensive stance coupled with a message that the complaint is not being dismissed offhand. In a similar vein, a group therapist who was accused of being a "phony" responded, "How can you judge me a phony if you didn't give yourself a chance to get to know me?"

Silences on the part of individual group members should not be confused with withdrawal from group participation. We have known many individuals who, while refraining from talking during the sessions, nevertheless showed surprising gains from the group experience, probably due to their vicarious involvement in the process. In contrast, with individuals who are obviously refusing to participate, exploring the possible reasons for this behavior (i.e., not trusting the group, or feeling that one doesn't have anything worthwhile to say) is an appropriate strategy.

Monopolizers, people who talk too much, are an ever-present problem in therapy groups. Hopefully, they will be confronted by the other members early on. Should this not occur, it is the therapist's task to deal with their behavior. The following two approaches, used successively, usually work: 1) "Why are you permitting Jane to take so much of the group's time?" 2) If this fails, a direct appeal to Jane should follow: "What you have to say is obviously important—but others also need a chance to talk."

Storytelling refers to a subtle defensive behavior akin to pseudo-disclosure—being devoid of feeling and dealing in obsessive detail with outside events. For instance, Carol, who began to complain about her mother, proceeded to elaborate and soon found herself rendering her mother's life story. The female therapist commented: "You seem to be talking more about your mother right now than about yourself. How are you affected by her behavior?" Shortly after, inviting feedback from the group, which had let Carol hold the stage for a long time, she added: "What is the group's impression of Carol's difficulty in dealing with her mother? Does this spark any feelings in some of you?"

In instances of unprovoked and openly expressed hostile behavior toward a peer, where neither the victim nor the group appears able to deal with it effectively, the therapist might invite the members to tell how they were affected by what had happened. Without permitting this to lead to scapegoating, the hostile youth should be asked in turn what he or she really wants from the group. (It might well emerge that the attack was a defense against becoming intimate.)

Earlier in this chapter we listed some typical group resistances such as testing operations and diversionary tactics. It is best to acknowledge to the group that while resistances always fill a need, they do not always require immediate handling. Thus, there might be moments when clowning in the face of a truly painful theme calls for a direct confrontation. At other times, this same clowning behavior might be accepted with the statement, "Perhaps the group is not yet ready to tackle such a charged issue." If bickering is used as a diversion in a group, the therapist could say: "It seems as though the group is letting chaos take over at times, so as to get rid of too much emotion."

Negative transference manifestations and scapegoating, in contrast, should be dealt with as they occur lest they poison the therapeutic climate. In instances of negative transference a mere exploration of the reasons for the momentary dissatisfaction or anger suffices to restore at least a modicum of a therapeutic alliance. It is often useful to enlist the help of the group by saying: "It feels to me as though I did something to make you angry. Could you tell me what it was?" As for scapegoating, as elaborated elsewhere by Scheidlinger (1982), only after "first-aid" is administered to the victim does the therapist enlist the group's input regarding the *why* and *how* of the phenomenon. In scapegoating among adolescents, attacks on "babyish" peers usually reflect unacceptable wishes not to have to grow up; labeling someone as "dumb" may mean that the perpetrators saw in the victim their own fear of failing school; and, not unlike adults, scapegoating "queers" is usually a projection of one's own homosexual concerns.

In distinction from adult groups, where long silences usually lead to the uncovering of latent themes when "process" interpretations are invoked, adolescents get unduly anxious by group silences. The therapist is therefore advised to interrupt the silence by initiating a subject for discussion, relating some relevant information, or simply encouraging someone to begin by recognizing the understandable reluctance to being the first in "getting the ball rolling."

The Group Therapist: An Almost "Impossible" Role

The material presented so far has documented beyond doubt that, to say the least, working with adolescents in groups calls for both art and skill. It takes a virtual juggling act to maintain a therapeutic alliance in the face of the intricate "below-the-belly" kind of provocative testing and of group-level resistances likely to surface at any time. It is, furthermore, far from easy to avoid being pushed into the role of the real parent, or of other hated adults, and yet not behave like "one of the gang." A sense of humor—laughing *with* but not *at* the youngsters—is an enormous help.

The findings from a study of therapeutic factors in adolescent groups are instructive (Corder et al. 1981). From among the 12 hypothesized factors posited by Yalom (1975), a selected sample of adolescent group patients listed four therapeutic factors as having been most helpful to them:

1. Catharsis (in the sense of being able to say what was disturbing rather than holding it in, as well as learning how to express one's feelings).
2. Existential factors (learning to take ultimate responsibility for one's behavior).
3. Interpersonal learning (other members honestly saying what they think of one another).
4. Family reenactment (being in the group, in a sense, experienced as being in a big family, albeit a more accepting and understanding family).

It is noteworthy that the factor of insight was deemed by the sample as being the least helpful of the curative factors.

A Look at the Future

As more clinicians advocate expanded mental health services for youth (Jemerin and Phillips 1988), new opportunities for group treatment are bound to develop. In a study sponsored by the National Institute of Mental Health, Thompson and his associates (1986) found a significant increase in the use of adolescent group therapy in clinical settings. This was due in part to the pressure from third-party payers for less costly and more efficient intervention modalities.

There has been a marked rise in the training opportunities for prospective adolescent group workers during the last few years, together with numerous publications, including three monographs (Azima and Richmond 1988; Rose and Edelson 1987; Siepker and Kandaras 1985). Comparing this figure with the total of only five books on the group treatment of adolescents that appeared during the previous 15 years, the future of group psychotherapy for adolescents is promising.

References

Adelson J, Doehrman MJ: The psychodynamic approach to adolescence, in Handbook of Adolescent Psychotherapy. Edited by Adelson J. New York, Wiley-Interscience, 1980, pp 99–116
Azima FJ: Transference-countertransference issues in group psychotherapy

for adolescents. International Journal of Child Psychotherapy 1:51–70, 1972

Azima FJ, Richmond L (eds): Adolescent Group Psychotherapy: Contemporary Issues. Madison, CT, International Universities Press, 1988

Blos P: Intensive psychotherapy in relation to the various phases of the adolescent period. Am J Orthopsychiatry 32:901–910, 1962

Blos P: The Adolescent Passage: Developmental Issues. New York, International Universities Press, 1979

Corder B, Whiteside L, Haizlip T: A study of curative factors in group psychotherapy with adolescents. Int J Group Psychother 31:345–354, 1981

Davis F, Lohr N: Special problems with the use of co-therapists in group psychotherapy. Int J Group Psychother 21:943–958, 1971

Freud A: Adolescence. Psychoanal Study Child 13:255–278, 1958

Gardner R: Psychotherapy With Adolescents. Cresskill, NJ, Creative Therapeutics, 1988

Garland JA, Jones HE, Kolodny RI: A model for stages in development in social work groups, in Explorations in Group Work: Essays in Theory and Practice. Edited by Bernstein S. Boston, MA, Milford House, 1973, pp 21–30

Jemerin J, Phillips I: Changes in inpatient child psychiatry: consequences and recommendations. J Am Acad Child Adolesc Psychiatry 27:397–403, 1988

MacLennan B, Felsenfeld N: Group Counseling and Psychotherapy With Adolescents. New York, Columbia University Press, 1968

Phelan J: Parent, teacher or analyst: the adolescent group therapist's trilemma. Int J Group Psychother 24:238–244, 1974

Rachman A: Group psychotherapy in treating the adolescent identity crisis. International Journal of Child Psychotherapy 1:97–119, 1972

Redl F: When We Deal With Children. Glencoe, IL, Free Press, 1966

Rose, SD, Edelson JL: Working With Children and Adolescents in Groups. San Francisco, CA, Jossey-Bass, 1987

Rosenthal L: Some dynamics of resistance and therapeutic management in adolescent group therapy. Psychoanal Rev 58:353–366, 1971

Scheidlinger S: Focus on Group Psychotherapy. New York, International Universities Press, 1982

Scheidlinger S: Group treatment of adolescents: an overview. Am J Orthopsychiatry 55:102–111, 1985

Siepker BB, Kandaras CS (eds): Group Therapy With Children and Adolescents. New York, Human Services Press, 1985

Slavson S: Analytic Group Psychotherapy. New York, Columbia University Press, 1950

Sullivan H: The Interpersonal Theory of Psychiatry. New York, WW Norton, 1953

Thompson JW, Rosenstein M, Milazzo-Sayre L, et al: Psychiatric services to adolescents: 1970–1980. Hosp Community Psychiatry 37:584–590, 1986

Yalom I: The Theory and Practice of Group Psychotherapy. New York, Basic Books, 1975

Specific Disorders and Their Treatment

Psychotherapy of Adolescents With Attention-Deficit Disorder

ROBERT L. HENDREN, D.O.

Chapter 7

Psychotherapy of Adolescents With Attention-Deficit Disorder

*T*he persistence of attention-deficit disorder[1] (ADD) into adolescence and young adulthood can be understood and successfully managed through an appreciation of the multidimensional factors involved in its pathogenesis and sequelae. Biological, psychological, and social factors interact with environmental and developmental factors to ameliorate or worsen the associated symptoms. In this chapter these factors will be reviewed and an effective psychotherapeutic management program for the adolescent with ADD will be described.

ADD is not outgrown in adolescence. While an estimated 3% of school-age children (primarily boys) are reported to have ADD (American Psychiatric Association 1987), longitudinal follow-up studies indicate that many of these children continue to experience problem behavior in adolescence and young adulthood (Hechtman et al. 1984a, 1984b; Hoy et al. 1978; Weiss 1985; Weiss et al. 1971). Although the percentage of ad-

---

[1]Attention deficit disorder (ADD), attention-deficit hyperactivity disorder (ADHD), and hyperactivity are used interchangeably in much of the literature and will be used synonymously in this chapter.

olescents who continue to experience symptoms varies to some extent from study to study, an average of one-third of former ADD children continue to show clear evidence of ADD as adolescents (Klee and Garfinkle 1983).

In the past the hyperactive syndrome was believed to be outgrown. Maturation of the central nervous system (CNS), along with improved methods of self-control, was suggested as a reason for the diminishing overactivity noted in adolescence. This diminishing overactivity was erroneously believed to represent resolution of the syndrome. However, a series of follow-up studies revealed a different natural history for the disorder. Although excess activity becomes less prominent, poor sociability (Loney et al. 1981), low self-esteem (Hoy et al. 1978), and impulsivity and distractibility (Waddell 1984) continue to be significant problems for adolescents who were found to have ADD in childhood. In a study group of hyperactive children initially identified during elementary school, the primary complaints at 13 years of age were poor academic performance, immaturity, and an inability to sustain goals (Weiss et al. 1971, 1978). The motor restlessness that was present initially was no longer the chief complaint. By age 19, hyperactive subjects continued to show greater impairment in academic and social abilities than did control subjects. Other follow-up studies supported the findings that physical hyperactivity diminishes during adolescence, but social, behavioral, and academic problems continue in subjects formerly with childhood hyperactivity (Ackerman et al. 1977).

Biological Factors

In familial studies of ADD children an increased risk of psychiatric disorders was found in the biological mothers and fathers of these children. Morrison and Stewart (1971) reported that approximately 30% of the "hyperactive" children in their studies had a formerly hyperactive parent. Approximately 70% of these parents presented with current psychiatric diagnoses, including alcoholism, sociopathy, depression, and psychoses. In his study of hyperactive children, Cantwell (1972) found that 10% of the parents were themselves hyperactive as children. All of these parents were experiencing psychiatric problems at the time of the study.

Hormonal differences are reported among groups of patients with ADD who respond to stimulant medications, suggesting the presence of a psychobiological defect (Cantwell 1983). In addition, there is preliminary evidence to suggest that ADD patients who later become delinquent have larger brain evoked potentials as children and smaller evoked potentials as adolescents when compared with healthy control subjects (Cantwell 1983).

These studies, when coupled with the response of ADD symptomatology to psychotropic medications, support a biological and, in part, inherited propensity to ADD. Further studies are necessary to delineate the psychobiological mechanisms responsible and to differentiate the influences of family environment from genetic heritability. Nevertheless, it seems clear that biological factors create a greater vulnerability to the development of ADD and that these factors are as influential in adolescence as they are in childhood.

Psychological Factors

Attention-deficit–disordered children as adolescents continue to demonstrate impulsivity, recklessness, and distractibility (Waddell 1984). In addition, they have little self-confidence, anticipate failure, avoid social participation, possess little self-discipline, and have fewer interpersonal interactions than do healthy control subjects. Overall, their self-esteem is low and they tend to see themselves as inadequate persons who are dissatisfied with their own behavior and morality, and who expect very little from the future. Weiss and her colleagues (Weiss 1985) noted marked sadness and depression among their adolescent hyperactive group. Others noted that hyperactive learning-disabled boys have significantly more problems with self-confidence than do normative learning-disabled boys or healthy control subjects (Ackerman et al. 1977). Fifteen percent of Mendelson and coworkers' (1971) sample of hyperactive boys had talked of or had attempted suicide.

Certain adolescents and young adults who have exhibited symptoms of ADD are more likely to develop characterological disorders, antisocial personality traits, and even psychotic disturbances than are healthy control subjects (Hechtman et al. 1984a, 1984b; Weiss 1985). However, prospective studies suggest that antisocial problems are less common than previously thought, particularly when hyperactive individuals are compared with control subjects matched for socioeconomic level and IQ (Hechtman et al. 1981).

Satterfield and colleagues (1982) found a dramatic increase in both arrests and repeated arrests in a hyperactive group when compared with matched control subjects. However, the increased arrests came largely from a group of hyperactive adolescents who had refused follow-up. Thus, factors that result in poor follow-up, such as a chaotic home environment or uncooperative parents, may have been responsible in part for the increased trouble with the law.

Research that has looked carefully at the characteristics of adolescents with a history of ADD who are experiencing problems reveals that predictors making the greatest contribution to these problems at follow-up are lower socioeconomic status, less controlling fathers, and, most importantly, aggressive symptomatology noted in childhood (Milich and Loney 1979). An indicator of aggressivity at referral (control deficits, negative affect, aggressive interpersonal behavior) was the single best predictor at follow-up for both aggression and hyperactivity factors obtained at follow-up. These findings suggest that adolescent behavioral outcome is unrelated to the degree of hyperactive symptomatology, but is related to so-called secondary symptoms of hyperactivity, especially the level of aggression demonstrated by the child as well as family interactions related to aggression.

Social Factors

During adolescence the ADD child is likely to experience social and academic problems due in large part to the psychological and behavioral problems discussed previously. In a series of follow-up studies Weiss and her colleagues (Hechtman 1984a, 1984b; Hoy et al. 1978; Weiss et al. 1971) noted that the primary complaints of parents of ADD adolescents were poor academic performance, immaturity, and an inability to sustain goals. Seventy percent of this follow-up sample had repeated grades, 10% were in special classes, and 5% had been expelled from school. The 20% who were functioning well academically differed from the others only on the basis of a higher IQ. Ackerman et al. (1977) found that 57% of the individuals in their hyperactive learning-disabled sample repeated one or more grades in school, compared with only 16% of healthy control subjects. Compared to an average drop-out rate of only 4%, Huessy et al. (1974) found that 21% of their follow-up sample of 75 hyperactive adolescents had dropped out of school.

The behavioral problems of ADD adolescents are found to move from the classroom into society at large. Mendelson et al. (1971) found that 59% of their sample had some contact with the police: 17% had been found to carry weapons, 15% had set one or more fires, and nearly 33% had threatened, at least once, to kill their parents. Other studies have also found that ADD adolescents are more likely to have serious social adjustment problems, including delinquency, serious acting-out behavior, and problems with school authorities (Ackerman et al. 1977). In addition, teacher and parent ratings suggest poorer levels of peer acceptance for ADD adolescents compared with those for healthy control subjects (Riddle and Rapoport 1976).

From the studies of ADD adolescents to date, it is not possible to determine how much of their social difficulty is due to the ADD per se and how much is due to the results of having a disorder that makes it difficult for them to fit into their social context. It is likely that these children who have difficulty attending to their parents, teachers, and peers experience a feeling of not fitting in with their family, their classroom, or their peer group. This sense of alienation and the resulting low self-esteem may lead them to less socially acceptable behaviors and to interacting with other peers who are on the "fringe" of society. None of the studies reviewed have specifically examined this effect on adolescent functioning. However, Weiss and colleagues (1978) found that work performance outside the classroom is less problematic for subjects with a history of ADD. Employer ratings of hyperactive and control subjects did not differ on descriptions of such behaviors as fulfillment of work assignments, getting along with coworkers, and independent work. The authors suggest that this improved performance in the work setting is due to the greater amount of freedom to choose employers, coworkers, and tasks.

Outcome and Sequelae of Treated and Untreated ADD Adolescents

As the studies above indicate, there is fairly consistent evidence that ADD subjects experience significant difficulties in adolescence and young adulthood. Unfortunately, there are few studies demonstrating that any treatments are effective in either preventing these difficulties or reducing their effects once they have begun (Milich and Loney 1979). Weiss and colleagues (1975) found that hyperactive subjects treated with methylphenidate for 3 to 5 years in childhood were not significantly different in adolescence from hyperactive children receiving chlorpromazine or those receiving no pharmacotherapy at all on measures of delinquency, emotional adjustment, hyperactivity, or school performance. Charles and

Schain (1981) found no differences between hyperactive children receiving either long-term or short-term methylphenidate treatment on behavioral ratings at home and at school. Similarly, Loney and colleagues (1981) found a continuation of ADD symptomatology, including social and academic problems, in their carefully controlled follow-up of children who received long-term stimulant drug therapy.

Studies of ADD children receiving multiple therapies, including medication and adjunctive therapies, also failed to show clear benefits from treatment (Feldman et al. 1979; Satterfield et al. 1982).

Many clinicians and researchers are surprised by the lack of research findings demonstrating long-term treatment benefits, since stimulant medications are symptomatically effective and appear to produce some long-term advantages for hyperactive children treated with them. Many of the follow-up studies of hyperactive children were reported a number of years ago, and there are few recent studies that reflect the greater understanding of the multiple factors involved in the etiology and treatment of ADD and the relationship of these to outcome of the disorder. Earlier in this chapter several studies were reviewed that suggest that outcome may be more related to measures of family pathology, low IQ, low socioeconomic status, drug response, and aggressivity at referral than to hyperactivity per se. Hechtman and colleagues (1984b) found that compared with untreated hyperactive children, stimulant-treated ADD children had fewer car accidents, viewed their childhood more positively, and had better social skills and self-esteem. Perhaps further exploration of factors such as these in a sample of individuals treated recently will reveal clearer benefits from stimulant treatment.

Management

Recognition and Diagnosis

During adolescence the behavioral overactivity present in children with ADD becomes less prevalent. This has, at times, caused clinicians to assume that ADD is outgrown in adolescence. If the adolescent is experiencing a persistence of ADD, the most likely presenting complaint will be academic underachievement and/or antisocial behavior (Wender 1983). Some young people with previously undiagnosed ADD may present for the first time in adolescence with a history of behavior and attention problems that have worsened with the stress of adolescence. Thus, it is important to gather a complete history of academic functioning and behavior during the elementary school years from every adolescent who presents with school problems or acting-out behavior.

The diagnosis of ADD can be guided through the use of the DSM-III (American Psychiatric Association 1980) and DSM-III-R (APA 1987) criteria. In DSM-III the hallmarks of ADD are short attention span and impulsivity, which are present with or without hyperactivity. The DSM-III-R has only one ADD diagnosis, that of attention-deficit hyperactivity disorder (ADHD), and it is no longer possible to identify the presence or absence of hyperactivity. This seems unfortunate because hyperactive behavior tends to decrease in adolescence and emphasis on this symptom may cause one to overlook the diagnostic possibility of ADD in an adolescent in whom hyperactivity is less prominent. DSM-III-R also includes a larger symptom list to describe the disorder (Table 7-1). When assessing an adolescent, a careful review of the symptoms related to a short attention span and impulsivity is helpful in recognizing residual ADD.

Medication

If a complete assessment suggests the presence of ADD, pharmacological treatment should be considered. This assessment is especially important if previous stimulant medication has been tried and discontinued, even if apparently unsuccessfully. Because response cannot be predicted in advance, a stimulant medication trial should be arranged (Table 7-2). An effective method for this is to have someone serve as a symptom rater who is unaware of the drug or the dosage used (Kutcher 1986; Varley 1983). This method provides objective data about the potential value of pharmacological intervention and allows for clinical titration of the drug effect that balances behavioral control against overmedication and side effects.

Sixty percent to 85% of school-age ADD children benefit from treatment with stimulation medication (Cantwell 1980). Several studies (Kutcher 1986; Safer 1975; Varley 1983) provide evidence that stimulants are effective in the treatment of adolescents with ADD. There has been no evidence of the previously postulated excitatory response to stimulants at puberty. Klorman and colleagues (1987) studied 19 adolescents with a childhood history of ADD using a double-blind, crossover trial involving 3 weeks each of methylphenidate (40 mg/day) and placebo.

Table 7-1.   DSM-III-R diagnostic criteria for attention-deficit hyperactivity disorder

Note: Consider a criterion met only if the behavior is considerably more frequent than that of most people of the same mental age.

A. A disturbance of at least 6 months, during which at least eight of the following are present:

   (1) Often fidgets with hands or feet or squirms in seat (in adolescents, may be limited to subjective feelings of restlessness).
   (2) Has difficulty remaining seated when required to do so.
   (3) Is easily distracted by extraneous stimuli.
   (4) Has difficulty awaiting turn in games or group situations.
   (5) Often blurts out answers to questions before they have been completed.
   (6) Has difficulty following through on instructions from others (not due to oppositional behavior or failure of comprehension), e.g., fails to finish chores.
   (7) Has difficulty sustaining attention in tasks or play activities.
   (8) Often shifts from one uncompleted activity to another.
   (9) Has difficulty playing quietly.
   (10) Often talks excessively.
   (11) Often interrupts or intrudes on others, e.g., butts into other children's games.
   (12) Often does not seem to listen to what is being said to him or her.
   (13) Often loses things necessary for tasks or activities at school or at home (e.g., toys, pencils, books, assignments).

B. Onset before the age of 7.

C. Does not meet the criteria for a pervasive developmental disorder.

Source. Reprinted from American Psychiatric Association: *Diagnostic and Statistical Manual of Mental Disorders, 3rd Edition, Revised.* Washington, DC, APA, 1987, p. 52, with permission of the APA. Copyright 1987.

Parent and teacher ratings reported significant reductions of inattentiveness and overactivity and, to some extent, of disobedience. Thus, while the majority of follow-up studies have yet to demonstrate long-term benefits from stimulant treatment of ADD, symptomatic improvement is clear in treated adolescents. Reasons that stimulant medication may be judged ineffective in adolescents with ADD include 1) a dosage level inappropriate to accommodate the adolescent's continued growth, 2) noncompliance, or 3) an inadequate trial period.

While there has been some concern that adolescents treated with

Table 7-2.   Stimulants used in the treatment of attention-deficit disorder

Drug and dosage
Methylphenidate (Ritalin)
   0.3–1.5 mg/kg   10–50 mg/day
Dextroamphetamine sulfate (Dexedrine)
   0.3–1.5 mg/kg   2.5–40 mg/day
Magnesium pemoline (Cylert)
   0.5–3.0 mg/kg   37.3–112.5 mg/day

Medical management
Weight and height recorded every 2 weeks—more frequently if weight loss occurs.

Side effects
Decreased appetite, sleep disturbance, possible decreased growth, palpitations, tachycardia, hypertension.

Risk of discontinuance
Return of impulsivity, inattention, and hyperactivity; possible increase in social and behavioral problems.

---

stimulant medication may be at risk for substance abuse, follow-up research has not supported this possibility (Hechtman et al. 1984b). In fact, Loney and coworkers (1981) found that a positive response to methylphenidate was associated with a lower probability of drug abuse. When prescribing medication to an ADD child or adolescent, it is important to explain clearly the purpose of the drug and emphasize that it is used as a medical treatment for a medical condition. If there is continued concern about the potential for abuse, one method to help decrease the likelihood of abuse by the ADD adolescent or his or her friends is to supply the methylphenidate in dated envelopes on a weekly basis with the request that parents return all empty envelopes and unused medication to the clinic pharmacy (Brown and Borden 1986). In instances where potential abuse is worrisome, other medications might be considered, rather than withhold treatment.

There are several reasons to consider medications other than stimulants in the treatment of adolescent ADD. Although stimulants are the traditional first-line drugs, almost 30% of children do not seem to respond to any of the stimulants (i.e., amphetamine, methylphenidate, or pemoline). In addition, some ADD adolescents are noted to become euphoric on the same dosages of stimulants that previously had no ill effects. The potential for abuse, as noted above, is yet another reason to consider medications other than stimulants (Rapoport 1986).

In one study (Gastfriend et al. 1984), desipramine (Table 7-3) was found to be effective in the treatment of 11 out of 12 adolescents with ADD. Inattention, impulsivity, and hyperactivity were reduced within 4 weeks, and the effect was sustained. Plasma desipramine levels for a given dose varied widely among patients. In an earlier double-blind, crossover comparison of desipramine with methylphenidate and clomipramine in ADD children, Garfinkle and colleagues (1983) found the tricyclic antidepressants to be more effective than placebo, but less so than methylphenidate. However, the maximum dosage of tricyclics was higher in the study by Gastfriend. In addition, a differential response was noted for both drug groups. Stimulants were more effective in controlling excessive motor behavior, and tricyclics were more effective in improving dysphoria. Relatively low dosages of desipramine (50 to 125 mg) have been shown to improve hyperactivity after only a few days of treatment (Donnelly et al. 1986).

Many ADD children dislike taking medication (Brown et al. 1987), and medication can provide an excellent battleground for struggles within the family. It should be recognized that it is not unusual for adolescents to deny that they have a medical problem or a need for medication. When

Table 7-3.   Desipramine in the treatment of attention-deficit disorder

Drug and dosage
Desipramine   5 mg/kg   50–250 mg/day

Medical management
Baseline ECG prior to initiation of treatment. Repeat ECG at dosage above 250 mg/day, or in the event of any change in cardiovascular status.

Side effects
Anticholinergic effects; prolongation of P-R, QRS complex, and Q-T intervals; blood pressure changes; gastrointestinal upset on abrupt discontinuation.

Risk of discontinuance
Gastrointestinal upset on abrupt discontinuation, with flu-like symptoms.
Return of impulsivity, inattention, and hyperactivity.
Return of aggressive behavior.

serious resistance is encountered, the physician should spend time further developing a therapeutic relationship with the adolescent and his family.

Despite the effectiveness of drug therapy in adolescent ADD, it is clear that additional modalities are required (Klorman et al. 1987). First, the extent of these patients' difficulties, reviewed in the early portion of this chapter, often requires behavioral, psychological, and educational interventions. Second, even with successful treatment, some adolescents refuse to continue treatment. Brown and colleagues (1987) found that compliance with psychotherapy was more likely to occur than was compliance with pharmacological treatment of ADD. This finding suggests that other psychotherapeutic approaches in addition to pharmacotherapy are essential to effective treatment of adolescents with ADD.

The following case study provides an example of medication management in the treatment of ADD children:

> Shane is a 13-year-old boy referred for psychiatric hospitalization as a result of longstanding behavioral problems. In the past year Shane was suspended from school twice, once for verbally abusing his teacher and the principal, and once for truancy. Shane's parents were divorced when he was 6 years old. His mother describes his behavior as having become progressively more difficult for her to control when his father disappeared after their divorce. When Shane was 9 years old the family doctor treated him with Ritalin. When he did not respond to 15 mg of Ritalin, the medication was discontinued. He saw a counselor twice when he was 10 years old, but Shane lost interest and stopped attending sessions. At the time of evaluation Shane appeared oppositional and mildly depressed, but denied any significant problems, in spite of his school suspension and problems at home.
>
> During Shane's brief hospitalization his teacher noted that he had difficulty attending to classwork and was easily distracted. On the hospital unit he also had difficulty attending to tasks and often intruded into the activities of others for brief periods. He participated in therapy with his psychotherapist, but was easily distracted. His treatment team decided to institute a trial of stimulant medication in addition to his program of individual, group, and family therapy. Conner's rating scales were completed by his mother, his teacher, and his primary mental health worker. Ritalin was started at 5 mg twice a day and gradually increased over 3 weeks to the maximally effective dosage of 30 mg per day. Conner's rating scales were completed twice a week and demonstrated significant improvement in his attention. His psychotherapist noted that he was less distractible and could talk about emotionally

arousing topics for a longer period of time. Shane's mother found him less oppositional, both in family therapy and on weekend passes at home. Other children in the psychiatric unit found him less intrusive, and he began to make friends. Shane's teacher developed a school program that included individual time with her. This individualized program was shared with the teacher at the school in his community.

After 6 weeks of hospitalization, Shane was discharged to his mother's home. He continued with weekly outpatient individual and family therapy. Ritalin was continued at 30 mg per day. At follow-up 6 months after discharge, Shane had not experienced any problems at school, his relationship with his mother had improved according to both Shane and his mother, and he was beginning to develop a group of friends. He continued regular psychotherapy throughout the period of follow-up.

Psychotherapy

There is little research regarding the benefits of the use of psychotherapeutic techniques with ADD adolescents. A few studies of the successful use of operant techniques in the treatment of ADD children have been reported, but there may also be some limitations (Brown and Borden 1986). These limitations include limited generalizability of the reinforced behavior and evidence that the reinforcing agent may divert the child's attention from the task at hand. Cognitive approaches to encourage feelings of self-control have been tried but are at best only partially successful (Brown and Borden 1986; Brown et al. 1987). Biofeedback has proven modestly effective in one study in improving certain measures of self-esteem in ADD adolescents (Omizo 1980).

The review of past and present research presented earlier in this chapter of the psychological and social factors associated with ADD in adolescence suggests that individual, family, and group psychotherapy should be of both short- and long-term benefit to adolescents with ADD. Many clinicians who treat ADD adolescents report that there are clear benefits from these therapeutic approaches. However, no research study clearly demonstrates these benefits. There are several possible reasons for this. First, psychotherapy outcome is difficult to measure. Alternatively, it is much easier to obtain valid and unconfounded results in medication studies. Second, ADD follow-up studies have not controlled for factors such as IQ, psychological mindedness, family dysfunction, and motivation. These factors affect psychotherapy response and may have led to the conclusion that psychotherapy does not have long-term benefits. Finally, measures of outcome such as school performance may not reflect the benefits from psychotherapy as accurately as would measures of social relatedness and self-esteem.

Psychotherapy with the ADD adolescent should address both the nature of the disorder and the results of it. The biological basis of ADD should be explained to and understood by the adolescent and his family. Misconceptions about "badness," "oppositionalness," or "craziness" as the source of ADD should be explored. As noted previously, the self-esteem of these adolescents is very poor, and cognitive techniques may prove useful in elucidating assumptions and distortions that lead to depressive feelings. A supportive relationship with a psychotherapist can help the adolescent with ADD feel more accepted and less alienated from his or her social environment. This in turn may keep the adolescent from drifting into a group of antisocial peers bonded together by their feelings of alienation. Group therapy can also help the ADD adolescent find support from others, learn social skills outside the confinement of the classroom, and learn to express to others uncomfortable feelings that may otherwise be kept pent up. Supportive and cognitive psychotherapy and group experiences can also reveal more effective and socially acceptable ways to express aggressive and angry feelings.

Family sessions can encourage family members to support the ADD adolescent. For many families, education and support will be sufficient. However, for others, parental psychopathology and pathological family dynamics will need to be addressed with more intense psychotherapeutic intervention. When family change does not seem possible, the adolescent may need help in extricating himself from the pathological family interactions that result in his low self-esteem and his feelings of alienation. In a study by Weiss and coworkers (1971), adolescents who were hyperactive as children were asked, "What helped you the most during childhood?" The most common response was the identification with one parent who believed in the child's final success.

The following vignette illustrates how a combination of individual, family, and pharmacotherapy proved helpful to an adolescent with ADD:

> Described as very active as a baby, Barbara is a 16-year-old adopted daughter from a professional family. She began experiencing school and social problems at 9 years of age, consisting of short attention span, stealing money at home, and lying. The diagnosis of ADD was made,

but she received no medication. At 12 years of age she was seen by a child psychiatrist who prescribed Ritalin, which resulted in improved attention and behavior at school. However, over the next year, she experienced increasing depression and lowered self-esteem, and she began using marijuana heavily. After being caught using marijuana by the police, she was sent to an out-of-state boarding school. While there, her marijuana use increased, her school performance deteriorated, and eventually she was dismissed. She returned home and was referred for recommendation regarding inpatient treatment for substance abuse.

Barbara's parents were extremely angry with her. They had spent a great deal of money for her private school and she had once again disappointed them. Her mother was particularly resentful of the constant attention that Barbara received most of her life as a result of her behavioral problems and her physical attractiveness. Her father felt frustrated that in spite of his intellectual support and interest, Barbara continued to create embarrassing problems for their otherwise successful family. Barbara, a socially adept young woman, felt unaccepted by her family. She could not understand her repeating pattern of getting into trouble. Although she appeared untroubled on the surface, her self-esteem was in fact very low, and she spoke of deep feelings of sadness and unlovableness.

Individual therapy with Barbara focused on the origins of her low self-esteem, her tendency to make negative assumptions about how others were feeling about her, her feelings of alienation resulting from being adopted and having ADD, and her previously unconscious patterns of getting into trouble to keep her parents' attention. Family therapy focused on the dysfunctional relationship between the parents and their tendency to displace the focus of conflict onto Barbara, the parents' view of Barbara as dysfunctional and damaged, and both parents' tendency to become overly controlling when Barbara's behavior did not meet their expectations. In addition, Barbara was treated with long-acting methylphenidate, which she reported helped her to concentrate on her school work and to feel less irritable. A recreational drug abstinence contract was made with Barbara, and periodic urine drug screens were agreed upon.

Barbara and her family were seen regularly for 6 months and episodically as needed for another year. Barbara has remained drug free except for methylphenidate, her family conflicts have lessened dramatically, her school performance has improved, and she has not been in any noteworthy trouble in or out of school. She is presently applying to college and has a boyfriend and a group of "mainstream" friends.

School Programs

In recent years most school programs in major population centers have been well prepared to recognize ADD adolescents and provide for their special educational needs. The knowledgeable mental health professional can be a valuable collaborator in assuring that school-based programs are effective and helpful to the ADD adolescent. Improved communications, clear classroom structure, noise minimization, and cognitive behavior modification techniques have proven useful in improving attending behaviors (Shuck et al. 1987). The most successful programs motivate adolescents by focusing on areas of strengths. Special programs such as work-study or artistic enrichment programs may help the ADD adolescent feel successful in areas outside the confines of the classroom (Wender 1983).

Summary

Attention-deficit disorder in adolescence can be best understood and treated using a biopsychosocial model. It is important not only for the clinician to understand this multidetermined etiology but also for the adolescent and his or her family to appreciate that the roots of the disorder are not in oppositionality or "badness." While some ADD children seem to outgrow ADD, at least one-third show continued signs of ADD in adolescence, although there is a decrease in overactivity. While few outcome studies demonstrate clear long-term benefits from any treatment approach either alone or in combination with others, more current studies that focus on the multiple factors involved in outcome are beginning to demonstrate the benefits of treatment in certain groups of ADD adolescents. The combination of individual, group, family, and pharmacotherapy along with a school program that focuses on the adolescent's strengths is likely to prove most useful in helping the ADD adolescent successfully negotiate the combined stresses of adolescence and ADD.

References

Ackerman PT, Dykman RA, Peters JE: Teenage status of hyperactive and nonhyperactive learning disabled boys. Am J Orthopsychiatry 47:577–596, 1977

American Psychiatric Association: Diagnostic and Statistical Manual of Mental Disorders, 3rd Edition. Washington, DC, American Psychiatric Association, 1980

American Psychiatric Association: Diagnostic and Statistical Manual of Mental Disorders, 3rd Edition, Revised. Washington, DC, American Psychiatric Association, 1987

Brown RT, Borden KA: Hyperactivity at adolescence: some misconceptions and new directions. Journal of Clinical Child Psychology 15:194–209, 1986

Brown RT, Borden KA, Wynne ME, et al: Compliance with pharmacological and cognitive treatments for attention deficit disorder. J Am Acad Child Adolesc Psychiatry 26:521–526, 1987

Cantwell DP: Psychiatric illness in the families of hyperactive children. Arch Gen Psychiatry 27:414–417, 1972

Cantwell DP: A clinician's guide to the use of stimulant medication for the psychiatric disorders of children. J Dev Behav Pediatr 1:133–140, 1980

Cantwell DP: Attention deficit disorders. Clinical Update in Adolescent Psychiatry 1:2–7, 1983

Charles L, Schain R: A four year follow-up study of the effects of methylphenidate on the behavior and academic achievement of hyperactive children. J Abnorm Child Psychol 9:495–505, 1981

Donnelly M, Zametkin, A, Rapoport, JL, et al: Treatment of childhood hyperactivity with desipramine: plasma drug concentration, cardiovascular effects, plasma and urinary catecholamine levels and clinical response. Clin Pharmacol Ther 39:72–81, 1986

Feldman S, Denhoff E, Denhoff J: Attentional disorders and related syndromes outcome in adolescence and young adult life, in Minimal Brain Dysfunction: A Developmental Approach. Edited by Denhoff E, Stern L. New York, Masson, 1979, pp 144–148

Garfinkle BD, Wender PH, Sloman L, et al: Tricyclic antidepressant and methylphenidate treatment of attention deficit disorder in children. J Am Acad Child Psychiatry 22:343–348, 1983

Gastfriend DR, Biederman J, Jellinek MS: Desipramine in the treatment of adolescents with attention deficit disorder. Am J Psychiatry 141:906–908, 1984

Hechtman L, Weiss G, Perlman T: Hyperactives as young adults: past and current antisocial behavior (stealing, drug abuse) and moral development. Psychopharmacol Bull 17:107–110, 1981

Hechtman L, Weiss G, Perlman T, et al: Hyperactives as young adults: initial predictors of adult outcome. J Am Acad Child Psychiatry 23:250–260, 1984a

Hechtman L, Weiss G, Perlman T: Young adult outcome of hyperactive children who received long-term stimulant treatment. J Am Acad Child Psychiatry 23:261–269, 1984b

Hoy E, Weiss G, Minde K, et al: The hyperactive child at adolescence: cognitive, emotional and social functioning. J Abnorm Child Psychol 6:311–324, 1978

Huessy H, Metoyer M, Townsend M: Eight–ten year follow-up of 84 children treated for behavioral disorder in rural Vermont. Series Paedopsychiatrica 40:230–235, 1974

Klee SH, Garfinkle BD: A comparison of residual and nonresidual attention deficit disorder in adolescence. The Psychiatric Hospital 14:167–170, 1983

Klorman R, Coons HW, Borgstedt AD: Effects of methylphenidate on adolescents with a childhood history of attention deficit disorder, I: clinical findings. J Am Acad Child Adolesc Psychiatry 26:363–367, 1987

Kutcher SP: Assessing and treating attention deficit disorder in adolescence—the clinical application of a single-case research design. Br J Psychiatry 149:710–715, 1986

Loney J, Kramer J, Milich RS: The hyperactive child grows up: predictors of symptoms, delinquency, and achievement at follow-up, in Psychosocial Aspects of Drug Treatment of Hyperactivity. Edited by Gadow KD, Loney J. Boulder, CO, Westview Press, 1981, pp 381–415

Mendelson W, Johnson N, Stewart M: Hyperactive children as teenagers: a follow-up study. J Nerv Ment Dis 153:273–279, 1971

Milich R, Loney J: The role of hyperactive and aggressive symptomatology in predicting outcome among hyperactive children. J Pediatr Psychol 4:93–112, 1979

Morrison J, Stewart M: A family study of hyperactive child syndrome. Biol Psychiatry 3:189–195, 1971

Omizo MM: The effects of biofeedback-induced relaxation training in hyperactive adolescent boys. J Psychol 105:131–138, 1980

Rapoport JL: Antidepressants in childhood, attention deficit disorder and obsessive-compulsive disorder. Psychosomatics (suppl) 27:30–36, 1986

Riddle KD, Rapoport JL: A 2 year follow-up of 72 hyperactive boys. J Nerv Ment Dis 162:126–134, 1976

Safer DJ, Allen RP: Stimulant drug treatment of hyperactive adolescents. Diseases of the Nervous System 36:434–457, 1975

Satterfield JH, Hoppe CM, Schell AM: A prospective study of delinquency in 110 adolescent boys with attention deficit disorder and 88 normal adolescent boys. Am J Psychiatry 139:795–798, 1982

Shuck A, Liddle M, Bigelow S: Classroom modifications for mainstreamed hyperactive adolescent students. Techniques: A Journal of Remedial Education and Counseling 3:27–35, 1987

Varley C: Effects of methylphenidate in adolescents with attention deficit disorder. J Am Acad Child Psychiatry 22:351–354, 1983

Waddell KJ: The self-concept and social adaptation of hyperactive children in adolescence. J Clin Child Psychol 13:50–55, 1984

Weiss G: Follow-up studies on outcome of hyperactive children. Psychopharmacol Bull 21:169–177, 1985

Weiss G, Minde K, Werry J, et al: Studies on the hyperactive child, VIII: five-year follow-up. Arch Gen Psychiatry 24:409–413, 1971

Weiss G, Hechtman L, Perlman T: Hyperactives as young adults: school, employer, and self-rating scales obtained during ten-year follow-up evaluation. Am J Orthopsychiatry 48:438–445, 1978

Wender EH: Hyperactivity in adolescence. J Adolesc Health Care 4:180–186, 1983

Chapter 8

Psychotherapy of Adolescents With Behavioral Disorders

RICHARD C. MAROHN, M.D.

Chapter 8

Psychotherapy of Adolescents With Behavioral Disorders

*T*wenty-five percent of the homicides, rapes, robberies, assaults, and arsons in this country are committed by persons under 18 years of age, even though this group comprises only 15% of the population (Marohn 1979, 1982; Zimring 1978). Half of the children in treatment present because of aggressive behavior (O'Donnell 1985), while childhood behavioral problems, such as aggressive conduct, stealing, truancy, lying, and drug use, predict later serious delinquency (Loeber and Stouthamer-Loeber 1987).

Behaviorally disordered children from the mental health system migrate to the correctional and juvenile justice systems as they become adolescents, because their violent behavior and their size frighten others and also make them more difficult to manage. Many disturbed adolescents in correctional facilities have been relocated there from therapeutic settings because of their behavior. Prisons must now function as treatment units for disturbed and violent adolescents (Lewis and Shanok 1976).

Psychiatric Aspects of Adolescent Behavioral Problems

Our society is preoccupied with unemployment, racism, poor schools, and poverty as causes of juvenile delinquency (Marohn 1979), and, as a

145

result, behavioral scientists, psychiatrists, and other clinicians are usually ignored when public policy is being formulated. Nonetheless, psychological factors are pertinent. Many adolescents use substances to soothe and regulate themselves (Marohn 1983). Violent death, a serious problem for impulsive adolescents (Marohn et al. 1982), is associated with alcohol use almost half of the time in the 15- to 19-year-old age group (Abel and Zeidenberg 1985).

Character structure emerges from adolescence. Adolescents have responded to increased tensions by experimenting with and developing new ways of coping. They attempt to integrate genitality into the personality and to modify their attachments to the parents of childhood. They increasingly emphasize peer relationships that assume important self-object functions. In the context of these experienced relationships, various narcissistic and libidinal claims and wishes are hindered; if these frustrations are tolerable and can be mastered, they are structured into the personality as functions that the adolescent now performs for himself or herself. What peers—same sex and opposite sex—and parents provide for adolescents become small accretions of psychic structure, and adolescents can now modulate and channel their urges, calm and soothe themselves, regulate their self-esteem, judge their performance realistically, plan how to fulfill their ambitions, and revere and respect important people without being swept away in crushes. The multiple infatuations of the fickle adolescent evolve into a youth's capacity for intimacy; this depends on a relatively intact and cohesive personality that has borne the threats of adolescent fragmentation, has integrated genital urges as part of the self rather than as foreign temptations, has begun to be regulated by one's own ideals and values rather than those of parents or society, and has experienced oneself as someone with a continuous past and prospective future. The interpersonal experiences of adolescence provide rich opportunities for the formation of competent psychological skills. The kinds of experiences that many adolescents have reflect, rather than cause, the internal shifts and growths that are occurring. For example, bad kids do not cause Johnny to become a delinquent (unless Johnny is a borderline who clings to whomever he can attach himself to), but Johnny's attraction for delinquent kids reflects something about his own inner psychological world, and he displays it, actualizes it, and practices it through his involvement in a gang. It is from this matrix of adolescent behavioral problems that adult personality disorders emerge.

Often, well-established behavioral patterns surface during adolescence. In our own research work, we described four parameters of non-psychotic adolescent delinquent behavior: impulsive, narcissistic, depressed borderline, and empty borderline (Marohn et al. 1979; Offer et al. 1979). Such work demonstrates the possibility of understanding, rather than simply describing, deviant adolescent behavior and shows that pervasive behavior patterns and psychodynamic formulations can be inferred, from which generalizations about assessment and treatment can be made.

Describing the individual psychodynamics of adolescent behavioral problems has a long history. Aichhorn (1925/1935, 1964) applied Freud's psychoanalytic discoveries to the "wayward youth" of Vienna and first described the idealizing transference and the role of primitive narcissism in such deviancy (Marohn 1977). Winnicott (1958, 1973) described the "antisocial tendency" of the delinquent to test destructively and to seek out a stable, structured relationship. Redl (1966) and colleagues (Redl and Wineman 1957) wrote repeatedly about the possibility of understanding impulsive behavior and reversing the process by providing auxiliary psychological functions through caregivers.

Additional work at the Illinois State Psychiatric Institute concentrated on the understanding and management of disturbed adolescent behavior. There is a close correlation between verbal threats of violence, damage to property, and assault on persons. Verbal threats, if unchecked, will escalate to physical assault (Marohn et al. 1980), whereas the verbal catharsis of angry feelings does not lead to further violent behavior (Curtiss et al. 1983; Ostrov et al. 1980). Many adolescents behave violently because they experience periods of traumatic overstimulation, often from strong wishes for affectionate contact that overwhelm them (Marohn 1974). Institutional riots result in part from such problems in tension regulation as well as from the tendency of property violence to intensify to personal violence (Marohn et al. 1973; Zinn and Miller 1978). Some adolescent violence expresses rage and destructiveness, often the rage of a primitive narcissistic personality. One tries to destroy an offending other, who fails to mirror or sustain the self or live up to idealized expectations; or, one tries to reconstitute a crumbling self by actively turning an injury into an assault and utilizing a familiar behavior pattern, destructiveness, to do so (Kohut 1972; Marohn 1977; Newman 1973).

Many have believed that depression and antisocial or aggressive behavior are diametrically opposed, that the aggressive individual is not suicidal, and that depressed individuals, having "internalized" their aggression, are not violent. Indeed, one tactic for treating depression involves helping patients express their anger, verbally or in an acceptable activity. However, we know that violent adolescents are often suicidal, and the violent, impulsive adolescent is at great risk for suicidal behavior and violent death (Marohn et al. 1982; Shaffer 1988).

The earlier a child behaves violently, the longer and more extensive the career of violence will be (Loeber and Stouthamer-Loeber 1987; Monahan 1981; Ryan 1986; Temple and Ladouceur 1986). In fact, the adult is usually not violent unless he or she was violent as a child or adolescent. The most reliable predictor of adult behavior is juvenile behavior (Wolfgang 1978).

Lewis and her colleagues (Lewis 1983; Lewis and Balla 1976; Lewis and Shanok 1976; Lewis et al. 1979, 1982, 1985; also qtd. in Adams 1987, p. 1) have described the neurological disorders and psychosis that underlie delinquency. Their work emphasizes the serious needs of the violent and incarcerated delinquent. However, the history of head injury and other abuse that these investigators describe also occurs in a family atmosphere that psychologically affects the developing child and adolescent. The prevalence of neurological "soft signs" in these subjects has not been replicated. Benedek et al. (1987) found a significantly lower incidence of psychosis in a population of adolescent murderers.

Abuse of alcohol and other substances, physical and sexual abuse, and family psychopathology have all been associated with adolescent psychopathology, or indicted as causal. Often, however, such actions are manifestations of underlying psychopathology rather than the causes. For example, although there is a correlation between substance abuse and adolescent delinquency, drug usage does not cause delinquency, but is rather another manifestation of the primary pathology (Kandel 1982). Many adolescents use alcohol and other substances to regulate, comfort, and soothe themselves because they cannot perform such psychological functions themselves and cannot employ others to assist them (Marohn 1983). Although 25% to 50% of adjudicated and institutionalized delinquents have been abused, this does not demonstrate conclusively that abuse leads to serious delinquency, because fewer than 20% of abused children become delinquent (Austin 1984).

Violent behavior is prevalent when culture and family condone it. As the child becomes an adolescent, violence is more acceptable (Bush 1985). Violent boys consider themselves healthy, whereas violent girls do not, and even treatment staff find something likable, or at least gratifying, in the violent patient (Offer et al. 1975). While association with a delinquent peer group does not *cause* serious delinquency, it is *predictive* of delinquency (Austin 1984); the adolescent's choice of peers usually illustrates his or her personality or basic psychological configurations.

Family violence results from diagnosable psychiatric illness, such as alcoholism, antisocial personality disorder, depression, or suicidal preoccupation (Bland and Orn 1986). Johnson and Szurek (1952) demonstrated that adolescents will enact the delinquent, but consciously disavowed, urges of their parents. Families that dismiss a child's temper tantrums, aggressive behavior, and noncompliance as "phases" will be confronted with further serious deviant behavior (O'Donnell 1985). Frequent and earlier separations from the parents seem to correlate with a more behaviorally aggressive child and adolescent rather than self-destructive progeny (Nielsen et al. 1985). Fire setting often occurs at a time of family stress and disintegration (Bumpass et al. 1974, 1983, 1985a, 1985b). Poor supervision at home, parental rejection of the child, lack of discipline and involvement by the parents, parental criminality and aggressiveness, and marital discord all predict future delinquency in the offspring (Loeber and Stouthamer-Loeber 1987).

When children serve exaggerated regulating or other sustaining functions for their parents, the degree of narcissistic injury parallels the kind experienced by the neglected child. Although many studies measure and attempt to correlate parental and adolescent histories and behavior in an effort to explain psychopathology, the crucial issue is how the child or adolescent *experiences* the parent and the parent's actions. The parent trying to be empathetic may not be experienced as such; the indifferent parent may be felt as vitally involved. Fundamental to the psychiatric explanation of all adolescent behavioral problems is the realization that all behavior has psychological meaning and can be understood psychodynamically (Marohn et al. 1980; Offer at al. 1979).

Treatment

Behaviorally disturbed adolescents are difficult to treat; their adjustment is brittle, and when threatened, they may become disruptive or even violent. Their hostility and negativism are inevitably repeated in their treatment, and, as a result, many therapists avoid this kind of patient (Marohn 1981). To treat this patient supportively is to evade this patient's violence and to fail him or her (Kernberg 1975). Whether rage is the result of a destructive inner drive (Kernberg 1974, 1979) or attendant on an inevitable narcissistic injury, it must be met by a confident and secure therapist (Marohn 1985). When adolescents do not have the psychological strength or support of friends or family to confront their pathology and violence in office therapy, they may need the relationships of the hospital or residential treatment staff (Easson 1969). The staff perform important sustaining functions for the psychologically defective, behaviorally disordered patient; they help to complete the adolescent's self. The psychotherapist can then focus on the material brought to him or her—not just verbal associations in the office session, but also the patient's behavioral associations on the treatment unit (Marohn et al. 1980).

Many of these behaviorally disordered adolescents are alexithymic and experience affect, but cannot use it as a signal of information. They have little awareness of an inner psychological world, cannot name affects or differentiate one affect from another, and often confuse thought, feeling, and deed. This kind of adolescent does not "act out" by externalizing an intrapsychic neurotic conflict. "Inside" and "outside" are explanations of the observer, not the patient's experience. To think is to feel is to do something; when these adolescents say that they did something because they "felt like it," they accurately describe their psychological state. The therapeutic task is to help these youthful patients accomplish an important adolescent transformation: to experience affect as part of themselves and to develop the capacity to manage affect and use it effectively as self-communication (Krystal 1974, 1975, 1978; Marohn 1983). When we try to engage these adolescents in a verbal treatment, we not only help them experience and learn about an inner psychological world but we facilitate certain maturational steps, converting motor behavior to verbal behavior.

Psychotherapy

Hostility and negativism are inherent in the psychotherapy of many adolescents and are not usually expressions of resistance. Instead, they lie at the very core of the psychopathology. For example, the negative transference (Marohn 1981) frequently develops in the therapy of the behaviorally disordered adolescent and should not be equated with the absence of a therapeutic alliance. Defiance is as much an indication of a bond as is obedience. In classical psychoanalytic theory the positive transference was viewed as an expression of the libidinal instinct, and the negative transference, an expression of the aggressive or destructive instinct. Because of the universality of human ambivalence, both transferences needed to be dealt with in treatment. It was thought that many treatments failed because the negative transference was never confronted and never dealt with. The negative transference could lead to the destruction of the therapy, for it would spill over and interfere with the establishment or maintenance of a therapeutic or working alliance—but, of course, so could the positive or erotic transference. Both negative and positive transferences can become resistances, and both can become problems in treating the adolescent inpatient or outpatient.

Sometimes, negativism is not a true transference, but more of a defense or a defense transference—an attempt to protect the adolescent from the emergence of positive transference feelings, the tendency to idealize the therapist, or expressions of a search for an idealized parent. Intrinsic to this tendency to idealize is also a tendency to deidealize or depreciate. Such deprecation may express a defense against the emergence of intense primitive longings for a perfect parent. Other such expressions of hostility may, indeed, represent the disillusionment that the adolescent has experienced time and time again—that the hoped-for parent has failed to materialize—and he or she may indeed be reexperiencing with the new therapist the combination of the two, the search for the wished-for parent and the expectation that this therapist, like other parents in the past, will fail him or her. Or, he or she may also have noticed some defect in this therapist and may experience the disillusionment that the idealized parent has once again failed to emerge. The competent therapist realizes that such negativism and hostility are expressions of the core pathology of the behaviorally disordered adolescent that indicate that an attachment does exist, an attachment that needs to be understood and worked through in the same way that a positive attachment needs to be worked through.

The behaviorally disordered or violent adolescent who is also suicidal presents complex problems in management and psychotherapy. As mentioned above, the therapist can no longer assume that the aggressive or delinquent adolescent is not at the same time depressed or suicidal. Increasingly, we recognize the interplay between violence toward self and toward others. It is important, therefore, for the psychotherapist not to be lulled into complacency when the adolescent's aggressivity diminishes or his or her depression lifts.

Impulsivity may be the underlying trait that causes such an adolescent to be a therapeutic challenge. The treatment program, then, is directed at assisting the patient to develop an internal regulating system; the therapist and the treatment milieu provide important selfobject functions, which, through transference interpretation, eventually become part of the patient's own psychological competence. Often, an inpatient milieu or psychopharmacological intervention may in fact be required to facilitate such structuralization.

An interesting clinical experience was described by Offenkrantz and colleagues (1978–1979) in their work with a group of heroin addicts, murderers, prostitutes, and suicide attempters who had been so exploited and deprived by their parents that they were incapable of empathic contact or tenderness. This group of individuals would often prefer to kill themselves rather than become aware that their parents considered them expendable and disposable (Tobin 1976). Here, suicide is being used by the impulsive individual to defend against narcissistic rage against the abusive parent.

In any psychotherapy the therapist is experienced as a real object and a transference object. The therapist of the adolescent is an important real-life person who facilitates important developmental change. Furthermore, the adolescent's therapist employs interventions that resonate with the depths of his own adolescent self-maturation (Marohn 1985). The therapist's self-esteem and self-assertiveness come to the fore; his therapeutic ambition moves him onward; his creativity shows itself in the way in which he expresses himself, and in what he expresses; his therapeutic and interpretive activity displays to the patient his inner self that moves in stride with his therapeutic aims. To be firm in the face of demands, devaluation, and depreciation and to interpret rather than gratify transference wishes and pleas is the work of a secure, confident, and unmovable therapeutic agent. Many charismatic figures work with adolescents, capable of being idealized and capable of establishing important narcissistic bonding, without, however, helping these adolescents develop their own psychological skills. At the other end of the spectrum are insecure, ambivalent, and defensive people who cannot engage the adolescent in any kind of relationship. The ideal road is that of the confident and secure therapist who does not assault his patients with his own grandiosity, but who shows initiative and assertiveness as he expresses his well-defined and securely held therapeutic aims.

Medication can be readily integrated into such a milieu and psychotherapy approach, not only for the physiological indications in certain situations but also to facilitate pacifying and organizing the patient's inner psychological world. Physical restraints, patient holding, and seclusion rooms can also be part of the therapeutic armamentarium in working with the hospitalized adolescent (Bornstein 1985; Marohn et al. 1980; Tomkiewicz 1984).

A careful diagnostic evaluation initiates the successful treatment of the behaviorally disordered adolescent. The prevalent psychiatric condition, for example, a bipolar affective disorder or a narcissistic behavior disorder, is the focus of the treatment, not the behavior as such, and an integrated treatment approach of psychotherapy, psychopharmacology, and milieu is formulated. Careful supervision of the treatment staff and of the psychotherapist provides the sustenance needed to work with these difficult and demanding patients. There are no research or clinical data that justify the use of psychopharmacological agents alone in treating the violent adolescent, without appropriate psychosocial and behavioral interventions (O'Donnell 1985).

Hospital and Residential Treatment

Patients experience their pathology in an autoplastic manner, as symptoms, or in an alloplastic way, as behavior. Developmentally, adolescents behave rather than experience symptoms, or affects, especially delinquents and behaviorally disordered adolescents. Because adolescents generally show their disturbances in their external behavior, rather than solely through traditional psychiatric symptoms such as psychosis and depression, psychiatrists and other mental health professionals who ignore delinquent and behaviorally disordered adolescents are missing, and failing, the vast bulk of disturbed teenagers.

The behavior of disturbed adolescents impinges on other patients, hospital staff, and the milieu, which must accommodate, change, or "push back." To "push back" is to reverse the externalization of the internal psychological world and produce an inner psychological distress—to understand the nature of the psychological deficit, to designate it, and to supply it or to help the patient develop competence or compensatory functions.

Limit setting is an important aspect of the hospital treatment of the behaviorally disordered adolescent. How well a therapist or staff member sets limits has something to do with how well or how poorly his or her own assertive tendencies have been transformed and integrated. The importance of setting limits in establishing internal psychological structure, controls, and coping mechanisms was repeatedly emphasized by Fritz Redl (Redl 1966; Redl and Wineman 1957). The external structure of the hospital milieu is eventually internalized as psychic structure by the adolescent (Marohn et al. 1980). A general goal of hospital or residential treatment of the behaviorally disordered adolescent is to convert acting-out behavior into some kind of internalized experience.

Clinical Examples

Nancy

Nancy is a 13-year-old who was hospitalized 2 years, and who, prior to admission, had had multiple group placements and psychiatric hospitalizations. She was violent at home, at school, and at other treatment facilities, stole frequently, truanted, and ran away. After admission she would assault staff without apparent precipitant, and it was only after several months that the sources of her rage became more clear. For awhile there was considerable pressure to think of her as having some kind of biological or hormonal imbalance, because it seemed that her disruptive and assaultive behavior was cyclical and not related to any apparent precipitant. However, the unit chief insisted that the staff hold to its philosophy that all behavior has meaning and can be understood psychologically, and that eventually, if the structure of the unit and of the daily program was maintained, the meaning of Nancy's behavior would become clear. Eventually, the sources of Nancy's rage were brought into the psychotherapy rather than discharged with other staff members.

Before she could talk openly in therapy sessions about her violent wishes and murderous urges that made her feel like "Hitler" and that she somehow felt were out of proportion to what they should be, she discussed them with ward staff and tried to organize some of these feelings and test out whether or not it would be appropriate to discuss these issues in psychotherapy. The ward staff were being used supportively.

Often, when Nancy became enraged, she would feel numb, a way of ridding herself of all intense affect, particularly rageful feelings. Eventually, she would rage at her therapist in sessions. She would scream at the therapist, and her speech would become garbled; she told her therapist that she wanted not simply to hurt her, but to strangle her. Staff recognized that Nancy used the ward staff and the therapist as selfobjects to complete herself and to provide psychological functions that she was not able to perform for herself. Conversely, she expected the therapist to use her also for narcissistic gain, and when the therapist recognized an accomplishment of Nancy's or seemed to be pleased that Nancy was making progress in psychotherapy, Nancy became enraged and felt that her gains had now been turned to "shit." The therapist met her rage by interpreting to her that Nancy felt that the therapist would not permit her to grow up and that she needed to kill the therapist in order to mature. Nancy regained her composure and agreed that she did feel that in order to grow, one had to kill the other person, that there was no way to have a relationship continue once one begins to grow, that people simply won't let one do that. Because the staff and therapist adhered to their treatment philosophy, Nancy's rage was confronted in the therapy rather than split off or suppressed.

Frank

Frank is a 15-year-old adolescent who came to treatment after several months in a hospital, where the therapist felt that he was a psychopathic individual who adhered to no value system and had no capacity to relate to others except for his own needs. His behavior was opportunistic and manipulative. He complained bitterly about the restrictions his parents placed on him that kept him from having fun and interfered with his peer experiences. Frank was involved in multiple delinquencies, including frequent runaways from home, serious school truancy, stealing money from his parents, taking the family car on a number of occasions without permission, sneaking out of the house during the early hours of the morning, using alcohol and drugs at home and outside of the home against his parents' wishes, selling marijuana and being arrested for it at school, driving a stolen car, driving without a license, and assaulting his older sister with a piece of furniture. All of these behaviors he saw in terms of his parents' refusal to give him freedom and autonomy.

It was clear after awhile that his protests of parental control were somewhat shallow, for he consistently provoked more and more parental control by his apparently rebellious behavior. Frank was attempting to ward off a serious depression, presumably related to the loss of nurturing and supportive relationships with both parents, who had heavily invested in his future as their only son. Any attempt on the part of each parent to try to understand his conflict or empathize with his struggles in achieving meaningful peer relationships was met with denial and rage. Similarly, when later on the therapist interpreted to him how his behavior, though by his claim designed to achieve autonomy, seemed to provoke more and more controlling responses by his parents, he angrily denied any such motivation. Gradually, however, the patient began saying that he had problems and could discuss these only with the therapist. Yet, at other moments, he would state quite openly that although he was pleased with his new school program and the restrictions it entailed, therapy had been of no help to him, despite his parents' insistence that it had been; and, indeed, he insisted that his parents were wasting their money. At the same time he, not defiantly, but quite comfortably, began traveling the substantial distance to the therapist's office by himself, no longer chauffeured by his parents. He enjoyed the freedom of exploration he found in taking public transportation, even in the depths of the winter. When spring approached, he talked about bringing his friends to a nearby park to show them the wonders of the city, at the same time indicating that he found that he could have fun, smoke marijuana, go to parties, and engage in what he felt were suitable adolescent activities without provoking parental control or causing parental discomfort. Indeed, although such attitudes had prompted a previous therapist to view him as a manipulator and a psychopath, this young man was beginning to appreciate the failings and unacceptability of his parents' value system, which he no longer needed either to idealize as omniscience or to depreciate as outmoded. Frank was now developing a belief system of his own. His rebellion indicated that a certain internal readjustment was occurring as he moved away from the sustaining and nurturing selfobject support of parental ties, replacing it with that of the therapist, and began to rely on his own values, comfortably and without apology.

In fact, he did bring his friends to a park in the neighborhood of the psychiatrist's office, and, as he described it with enthusiasm in a session a few days later, wondered if the therapist also was there in the park that same day. At the same time that he expected the therapist to be like him and be in the park at the same time, he denied the value of the sessions, felt that he and his parents were wasting time and money, and confronted the therapist with his explicit belief that "you don't help me." He insisted that all the changes he had made were changes of his own doing and asked for a 2- or 3-week control period away from treatment during which time he could demonstrate that he would continue to behave well without the need for therapy. The therapist's comments that he had improved were met with statements that he really did not care what the therapist thought; yet his behavior indicated an excitement and an interest in continuing the sessions.

Frank regularly depreciated and devalued the importance of the therapist, insisting not only that he did not need help, but that even if he did, the therapist could not help him. Nonetheless, he came regularly to treatment sessions, and it became clear that Frank was struggling to modify the intense narcissistic bonding to his parents, which was replicated in the treatment relationship. He believed that the therapist needed Frank for his own sense of well-being, and presumed that the therapist would demand of him some positive statements about the efficacy of the treatment. As a result, any comment about Frank's improvement would be met with the same disdain and disgust that he now heaped on his mother whenever she would attempt to praise him. Frank was struggling to transform his relationship with his therapist, and eventually did, having developed the capacity to take much greater responsibility for regulating his behavior and his life. Frank's negativism was the result of his need to modify his ties to his parental objects and, by transference, devalue and depreciate the therapist. His bonding with his parents was intensely narcissistic, and he could "free" himself only by negating the very nature of these attachments. The expectation of an exploitative narcissistic relationship with the therapist, as with the parents, was worked through and maturation achieved in termination. At those times when Frank would confront the therapist with the failure of therapy and the fact that he did not need any kind of treatment, the therapist would insist firmly that as far as the therapist was concerned, Frank desperately needed help, that he was unhappy, depressed, and angry, and that he would not improve without therapy. The therapist acknowledged that there was no way to force him into treatment, but noted that his stand was unequivocal—that there was nothing the patient could say or do to convince the therapist that he did not need help. The patient stopped arguing about the fact that he thought his parents were dragging him into treatment, and continued to come. Several months later, when the therapist indicated that he thought the patient had progressed to the point that he could choose to continue or discontinue treatment himself, the patient continued for another 6 months. Here, the therapist's taking a strong and unequivocal stand about the patient's pathology enabled the patient to continue to participate in treatment.

Conclusions

The relative tranquillity of young adulthood results from the maturation and development of self regulating systems. Such healthy development has complex biological, psychological, and social roots. Much can go awry, and the assessment of adolescent mental health and psychopathology is a consideration of relative deviation rather than one of clear-cut syndromes. Our perspective must be dynamic and systemic rather than classifying and sorting. Adolescent behavioral problems are complex, derived from psychological, biological, and sociocultural sources. Treating the behaviorally disordered adolescent is difficult, both in the office and in the hospital or treatment center.

References

Abel EL, Zeidenberg P: Age, alcohol and violent death: a postmortem study. J Stud Alcohol 46:228–231, 1985

Adams J: Clinical Psychiatric News, Dec 1987, pp 1, 16

Aichhorn A: Wayward Youth (1925). New York, Viking Press, 1935

Aichhorn A: Delinquency and Child Guidance—Selected Papers. New York, International Universities Press, 1964

Austin J: Statement before the Select Committee on Children, Youth, and Families, House of Representatives, U.S. Congress, May 18, 1984, in Youth and the Justice System: Can We Intervene Earlier? Washington, DC, U.S. Government Printing Office, 1984, pp 80–100

Benedek EP, Cornell DG, Staresina L: Violence and adolescence. Psychiatric Times, Oct 1987, pp 2, 4

Bland R, Orn H: Family violence and psychiatric disorder. Can J Psychiatry 31:129–137, 1986

Bornstein PE: The use of restraints on a general psychiatric unit. J Clin Psychiatry 46:175–178, 1985

Bumpass E, Via BM, Forgotson JH, et al: Graphs to facilitate the formation of a therapeutic alliance. Am J Psychother 28:500–516, 1974

Bumpass E, Fagelman FD, Brix RJ: Intervention with children who set fires. Am J Psychother 37:328–345, 1983

Bumpass E, Brix RJ, Preston D: A community based program for juvenile firesetters. Hosp Community Psychiatry 36:529–533, 1985a

Bumpass E, Brix RJ, Reichland RE: Triggering events, sequential feelings and firesetting behavior in children. J Am Acad Child Psychiatry 10:18, 1985b

Bush DM: Victimization at school and attitudes toward violence among early adolescents. Sociological Spectrum 5:173–190, 1985

Curtiss G, Rosenthal RH, Marohn RC, et al: Measuring delinquent behavior in inpatient treatment settings: revision and validation of the adolescent antisocial behavior checklist. J Am Acad Child Psychiatry 22:459–466, 1983

Easson WM: The Severely Disturbed Adolescent. New York, International Universities Press, 1969

Johnson AM, Szurek SA: The genesis of antisocial acting out in children and adults. Psychoanal Q 21:323–343, 1952

Kandel DB: Epidemiological and psychosocial perspectives on adolescent drug use. J Am Acad Child Psychiatry 21:328–347, 1982

Kernberg O: Further contributions to the treatment of narcissistic personalities. Int J Psychoanal 55:215–240, 1974

Kernberg O: Borderline Conditions and Pathological Narcissism. New York, Jason Aronson, 1975

Kernberg O: Psychoanalytic psychotherapy with borderline adolescents. Adolesc Psychiatry 7:294–321, 1979

Kohut H: Thoughts on narcissism and narcissistic rage. Psychoanal Study Child 27:360–400, 1972

Krystal H: The genetic development of affects and affect regression. Annual of Psychoanalysis 2:98–126, 1974

Krystal H: Affect tolerance. Annual of Psychoanalysis 3:179–219, 1975

Krystal H: Self-representation and the capacity for self-care. Annual of Psychoanalysis 6:209–246, 1978

Lewis DO: Neuropsychiatric vulnerabilities and violent juvenile delinquency. Psychiatr Clin N Am 6:707–714, 1983

Lewis DO, Balla D: Delinquency and Psychopathology. New York, Grune & Stratton, 1976

Lewis DO, Shanok SS: Medical histories of delinquent and nondelinquent children. Am J Psychiatry 134:1020–1025, 1976

Lewis DO, Shanok SS, Pincus JH, et al: Violent juvenile delinquents: psychiatric neurological, psychological and abuse factors. J Am Acad Child Psychiatry 18:307–319, 1979

Lewis DO, Pincus JH, Shanok SS, et al: Psychomotor epilepsy and violence in a group of incarcerated adolescent boys. Am J Psychiatry 139:882–887, 1982

Lewis DO, Moy E, Jackson LD, et al: Biopsychosocial characteristics of children who later murder: a prospective study. Am J Psychiatry 142:1161–1167, 1985

Loeber R, Stouthamer-Loeber M: The prediction of delinquency, in Handbook of Juvenile Delinquency. Edited by Quay HC. New York, John Wiley, 1987, pp 325–382

Marohn RC: Trauma and the delinquent. Adolesc Psychiatry 3:354–361, 1974

Marohn RC: The "juvenile imposter": some thoughts on narcissism and the delinquent. Adolesc Psychiatry 5:186–212, 1977

Marohn RC: A psychiatric overview of juvenile delinquency. Adolesc Psychiatry 7:425–432, 1979

Marohn RC: The negative transference in the treatment of juvenile delinquents. Annual of Psychoanalysis 9:21–42, 1981

Marohn RC: Adolescent violence: causes and treatment. J Am Acad Child Psychiatry 21:354–360, 1982

Marohn RC: Adolescent substance abuse: a problem of self soothing. Clinical Update in Adolescent Psychiatry, Vol 1, No 10, 1983

Marohn RC: Assertiveness in the treatment of juvenile delinquents. Psychiatric Annals 15:606–613, 1985

Marohn RC, Dalle-Molle D, Offer D, et al: A hospital riot: its determinants and implications for treatment. Am J Psychiatry 130:631–636, 1973

Marohn RC, Offer D, Ostrov E, et al: Four psychodynamic types of hospitalized juvenile delinquents. Adolesc Psychiatry 7:466–483, 1979

Marohn RC, Dalle-Molle D, McCarter E, et al: Juvenile Delinquents: Psychodynamic Assessment and Hospital Assessment. New York, Brunner/ Mazel, 1980

Marohn RC, Locke EM, Rosenthal R, et al: Juvenile delinquents and violent death. Adolesc Psychiatry 10:147–170, 1982

Monahan J: The Clinical Prediction of Violent Behavior. Rockville, MD, National Institute of Mental Health, 1981

Newman K: Some applications of concepts of the self to management of adolescents in the hospital. Bulletin of the Chicago Society of Adolescent Psychiatry, March 1973, pp 23–37

Nielsen G, Harrington L, Sack W, et al: A developmental study of aggression and self-destruction in adolescents who received residential treatment. International Journal of Offender Therapy and Comparative Criminology 29:211–226, 1985

O'Donnell DJ: Conduct disorders, in Diagnosis and Psychopharmacology of Childhood and Adolescent Disorders. Edited by Wiener JM. New York, John Wiley, 1985, pp 249–287

Offenkrantz W, Tobin A, Freedman R: An hypothesis about heroin addiction, murder, prostitution, and suicide: acting out parenting conflicts. Int J Psychoanal Psychother 7:602–608, 1978–1979

Offer D, Marohn RC, Ostrov E: Violence among hospitalized delinquents. Arch Gen Psychiatry 32:1180–1186, 1975

Offer D, Marohn RC, Ostrov E: The Psychological World of the Juvenile Delinquent. New York, Basic Books, 1979

Ostrov E, Marohn RC, Offer D, et al: The adolescent antisocial behavior check list. J Clin Psychol 36:594–601, 1980

Redl F: When We Deal With Children. New York, Free Press, 1966

Redl F, Wineman D: The Aggressive Child. Glencoe, IL, Free Press, 1957

Ryan G: Annotated bibliography: adolescent perpetrators of sexual molestation of children. Child Abuse Negl 10:125–131, 1986

Shaffer D: Personal, family factors in teen suicide identified. Clinical Psychiatric News, Feb 1988, p 2

Temple M, Ladouceur P: The alcohol-crime relationship as an age-specific phenomenon: a longitudinal study. Contemporary Drug Problems 13:89–115, 1986

Tobin A: Unpublished comments made at "Juvenile Delinquency: Contemporary Issues and Future Outlook," a conference sponsored by the American Society for Adolescent Psychiatry, Chicago, IL Jan 23–24, 1976

Tomkiewicz S: Violences et negligences envers les enfants et les adolescents dans les institutions [Violence and negligence to children and adolescents in institutions]. Child Abuse Negl 8:319–335

Winnicott DW: The antisocial tendency, in Collected Papers. New York, Basic Books, 1958, pp 306–315

Winnicott DW: Delinquency as a sign of hope. Adolesc Psychiatry 2:364–371, 1973

Wolfgang ME: An overview of research and violent behavior. Testimony before the House of Representatives Committee on Science and Technology, U.S. Congress, 1978

Zimring F: Background paper, in Confronting Youth Crime: Report of the Twentieth Century Fund Task Force on Sentencing Policy Toward Young Offenders. New York, Homes & Meyer, 1978, pp 27–120

Zinn LD, Miller DH: Riots on adolescent inpatient units. Journal National Association of Private Psychiatric Hospitals 9:42–51, 1978

Psychotherapy of Adolescents With Mood Disorders

JULES R. BEMPORAD, M.D.

Chapter 9

Psychotherapy of Adolescents With Mood Disorders

An essential component of the psychotherapeutic approach to the treatment of adolescent mood disorders is an understanding of the extent to which depression and elation are affected by and interact with the unique developmental characteristics of this stage of life.

There is uniform agreement that transient states of mild depression are a necessary and normal reaction to the losses and frustrations of everyday life. These temporary episodes of dysphoria demonstrate that we all have the ability to involve ourselves in our own environments and to grieve the loss of significant others or of ideals important to our sense of well-being. The capacity to bear and to overcome these reactions is a sign of good health. However, when depression is so profound as to impair functioning, or when individuals cannot realign their needs to compensate for their losses, or when trivial frustrations provoke inappropriately severe reactions, then the line between normalcy and psychopathology is crossed.

Alteration in mood can thus be conceived along a continuum from a normal, self-limited response to a narcissistic blow, to a crippling state of despair. This despair may be psychogenic in origin or may be the result of a physiological predisposition.

Defining Depression

Since the pioneering contributions of Bibring (1953), Sandler and Joffee (1965), and Arieti (1962), depression has been viewed as reaction to the loss of an internal or external factor necessary for the maintenance of self-esteem. Bibring saw the common core of depression in the ego's awareness of its inability to attain narcissistic aspirations, whether these involved relationships, environmental responses, or particular needs for achievement or admiration. He maintained that individuals prone to pathological depression include those who depend excessively on unreliable or external sources for a sense of well-being. Those individuals who appear more resilient are those whose basis for self-esteem is more firmly established. As such, they are relatively impervious to environmental vicissitudes.

Leff et al. (1970) found that occurrences that negatively influence one's concept of the self in relation to significant others often trigger depressive episodes. In support of this premise, Brown and Harris (1978) cite the case of a woman who became depressed upon learning that her husband had been unfaithful to her some years earlier. Although nothing tangible in her world was actually altered, her view of her husband, her marriage, and herself was clearly transformed. Ideals and values integral to her self-esteem were destroyed.

Jacobson (1961) further elaborates upon exaggerated alterations of adolescent mood. He maintains that adolescents must renounce their childhood sources of love and comfort, as well as former pleasures and pursuits. They must relate to new significant others and strongly rely on internal behavioral standards. They also, according to Jacobson, have to create new bases for their relationships, live by new values, develop new goals, and begin to consider the future. He states that "adolescence is life between a saddening farewell to childhood—i.e., to the self and the objects of the past—and a gradual, anxious-hopeful passing over the many barriers to the gates which permit entrance to the still unknown country of adulthood" (p. 165).

During this passage to adulthood, the adolescent's ego may sequentially side with the pressures of the id (resulting in stormy periods of sexual or aggressive acting out) or with the sanctions of the superego (resulting in shame, guilt, and feelings of inferiority). Eventually, the ego will master these pressures and consolidate a worthy sense of self. Along the way, however, external influences have an enormous effect on an ego weakened by rapid change.

Focusing on a more cognitive definition of depression, Easson (1977) speaks of "emancipation mourning"—that is, the coming to terms with reality in a more truthful and accurate way. As adolescents develop this ability, childhood denial can no longer quell painful realizations. Easson holds that there is a normal period of mourning over past cherished ideals or ambitions, which adolescents come to accept as unattainable. The fact that adolescents have the ability to critically assess themselves, while at the same time lacking the life experiences needed to moderate this ability, accounts for their often extreme reactions to seemingly trivial events. High school students who do poorly on a chemistry quiz may believe that they will never become doctors. Youngsters who are stood up on a date may be certain that they will never be able to establish intimate relationships. So despite obvious cognitive development, the realization that we all survive and grow regardless of immediate adversity has not yet come into play in the life of the adolescent. Life experiences are, at this point, rudimentary.

Defining depression within this broadened context sheds light on the high rate of mood disorders among adolescents and on the particular vulnerability of this population. It is during this time that relationships, values, aspirations and sense of self undergo rapid and sometimes radical change and reorganization—occurrences that are accompanied by characteristic mood extremes.

Comparing Adolescent and Adult Depression

The simultaneous occurrence of these numerous above-mentioned changes predisposes adolescents to an excessive reliance on external indicators of their worth and a consequent lability of mood. Periods of elation and depression, often to seemingly pathological degrees, rapidly occur and just as rapidly pass away.

Findings from a comparative study conducted by Csikszentmihalyi and Larson (1984) indicate that adolescents are less anchored in a familiar, middle-level, base-line state than are adults; they are more prone to swerving to one extreme or the other. In contrast to their elders, they are more likely to experience euphoria—to catch a glimpse of a world in which everything is perfect. However, they are also more vulnerable to sudden incursions of pain caused by unexpected events. Unlike adults, adolescents are less protected by the cumulation of experience.

Diagnostic and Therapeutic Considerations

Because rapid mood swings are so typical of adolescent behavior, difficulty often arises in determining when such states are pathological, and require clinical intervention, and when they can be left to resolve on their own. This lack of clarity is particularly true of depression. At the outset it may be impossible to determine if a depressed youngster is going through a normal reaction to some disappointment or if he or she is 1) presenting with an adjustment disorder with depressed mood, 2) suffering from a true clinical depression, or 3) exhibiting behavior indicative of the onset of bipolar disorder. An accurate diagnosis will entail taking an exhaustive developmental history, thoroughly examining family psychopathology, and carefully evaluating the level of current functioning.

The fact that symptoms are often short-lived also adds to the difficulty of making an accurate assessment. The exaggerated affect and the sense of urgency that frequently accompany rejection or disappointment make the dysphoric episode appear far more ominous than it actually is. Subsequent to a particular assessment, a seemingly despairing youngster may have totally recovered. He or she may have found a new source of fascination in which to invest his or her energies.

The film *Breaking Away* presents a charming illustration of such flightiness. The adolescent hero of the film drives his parents to distraction as he chases one ideal after another, falling into what appears to be complete despondency in between pursuits. Here, as in many TV sitcoms, the exaggerated travails of the adolescent are benign and comical.

In reality, however, dysphoric episodes in adolescents should always be taken seriously. Even when such episodes do not progress into actual depressive disorders, they may force youngsters who are in search of relief from pain to accept pathological solutions. These may include blatantly self-destructive behaviors such as drug abuse, promiscuity, or even suicidal gestures; or less obviously destructive anodynes such as entering into inappropriate relationships, giving up on career plans, or withdrawing from pleasurable and self-fulfilling activities.

These transient dysphoric episodes typically occur in healthy adolescents who, for the first time in their lives, are confronted with a major crisis. Such crises include being jilted by a boyfriend or girlfriend, failing to gain acceptance to a highly desired group such as an athletic team or honor society, or undergoing a transition that entails a loss of former status or security; this can be an event such as entering high school or college, or moving to a new location. In all such instances, adolescents believe that they do not fit in with peers, and miss their former sources of support.

Most adolescents with an adjustment disorder manage to realign their goals and compensate for threats to their emerging sense of self with minimal psychotherapeutic intervention. Psychotherapy here serves to put the immediate source of pain into perspective. It also helps youngsters to bear the despair or disillusionment that surround them and allows them to buy time until a more productive compensation can be found.

For those more vulnerable youngsters a more intensive and protracted form of therapy is indicated. In contrast to adolescents with an adjustment disorder, these patients present with poor coping abilities and histories of marginal functioning prior to their current episode. They have been so hampered by prior obstacles to growth that their sense of self and well-being is at risk of collapse with the slightest provocation. The cumulative effect of past fears and feelings of inferiority, coupled with the new and all-encompassing changes of adolescence, creates an insurmountable challenge for them.

Types of Adolescent Depression

These "true" depressions of adolescence have been described as two distinct clinical entities (Anthony 1975; Jacobson 1961). Although they have been labeled differently by various authors, their descriptions are similar. In keeping with distinctions made with adult depressed patients (Arieti 1962; Blatt 1974), this chapter will refer to these entities as "anaclitic" depression and "introjective" depression.

Anaclitic depression describes psychopathology that can be traced back to early stages of childhood. Adolescents with this type of depression have never truly separated psychologically from their nuclear families. They continue to require parental figures in order to feel secure and to ward off feelings of helplessness and abandonment. Marked dependency needs become prominent in periods of stress, as do shame and humiliation over the realization of these needs.

In contrast, introjective depression describes developmental problems that are believed to occur during or after the oedipal stage. Although adolescents with this type of depression have separated from their parents, they have internalized severe parental standards. As Anthony (1975) points out, the difficulty in this form of depression resides in a primitive superego, while in the anaclitic form the problem has more to do with the discrepancy between the ego and the ego ideal.

At the heart of both forms of depression is the inability to deal successfully with the psychosocial demands of adolescence as a result of prior maladaptive adjustment.

Anaclitic Depression

The clinical picture. Anaclitic depression occurs in those youngsters who are unable to dissociate themselves from the safety of preadolescent functioning. Although they cannot find real meaning from their own social, scholastic, or athletic abilities, they continue to use their achievements to ensure their security within the family system. Having never completed their developmental transition from latency in a satisfactory manner, they are unable to separate from family, and recoil in fear and shame at the new freedom offered by adolescent society. They are unprepared for the physiological changes occurring in their bodies, in their modes of thought, and in their patterns of social interaction. Although these youngsters may be quite bright, they are not at all "street smart." They typically rely on directions from parents or others as to how they should behave. They are both terrified and overwhelmed at having to exist without the security of adult structure and protection. Usually lacking in social skills, they are repeatedly teased or humiliated by peers.

The panic, bewilderment, and somatic symptoms so typical of this form of depression often obscure the underlying depression, thus making the diagnosis quite difficult. The sense of urgency and florid accessory symptoms may suggest an acute schizophrenic decompensation. The following clinical vignette describes an adolescent with this particular type of depression:

> Upon enrolling at the university, an 18-year-old college freshman became increasingly depressed. This young man had never had much exposure to dating or heterosexual relationships. Throughout school he was a straight-A student who shunned parties or other social events and relied exclusively on his academic record for self-esteem. This source of esteem was no longer sufficient, for his peers valued social life as much, if not more, than academics. He desperately missed the old security of home, where his parents rewarded his good grades and gave

him preferential treatment over his siblings. Stripped of their supportive value system, he viewed himself as woefully inadequate and socially inept. Despite a great desire to begin dating, whenever he attempted to engage a girl in conversation, he felt like he was making a fool of himself. This fear caused him to become paralyzed with anxiety. His mind would go blank.

When he came for therapy he was obsessed with the thought that he was homosexual and the belief that others thought so as well. This obsession appeared to be the transformation of a wish to be homosexual; because it was so much easier to talk to boys, he could thereby avoid the anxiety of heterosexual socializing. It was only after this almost delusional thinking subsided that he revealed his complete sense of failure and self-loathing because of his inability to function socially.

Therapeutic approaches. Therapy for anaclitically depressed adolescents involves a great deal of support and reparenting. The therapeutic setting should be perceived as a safe haven—a place where embarrassing fears and desires are accepted without critical comment. The first order of therapy is the acceptance of adolescents as they are, even if their environment continually reminds them of their deficiencies.

Second, symptom amelioration should be sought as rapidly as possible. This may involve pharmacological treatment. It may also necessitate environmental manipulation, such as suggesting that a college student who is socially tormented by his peers return home for weekends. Or, with the patient's approval, the therapist may contact parents in the hope of encouraging a more sustaining attitude on their part. The rapid resolution of presenting symptoms is also imperative if a correct diagnosis is to be made. Until the superimposed sense of panic and shame are mitigated, uncertainty as to the underlying illness will remain.

Once the acute symptoms have somewhat abated and a definitive diagnosis of depression established, therapy should explore areas of strength upon which to build a sense of worth. Some of these youngsters are poetic or artistic; others may excel in mathematics or science. Whatever their abilities, these should be maximized to provide feelings of security and satisfaction and to offer access points for entering into relationships with others, including the therapist. Discussions of science fiction or literature or physics or athletic events not only help to establish rapport with the therapist but also convey to struggling adolescents that they have something of value to communicate to others. Interests and feelings of worth can be enhanced by directing adolescents to clubs or groups focusing on their particular areas of expertise or interest. Hopefully, such an approach will enable them to value themselves and relieve the anxiety that socialization would otherwise engender.

In sum, therapy should serve as a means of enabling patients to enter adolescence at a more leisurely and relaxed pace, modifying the expectations and criticisms that are imposed upon them or that they impose upon themselves. Patience, support, and empathic acceptance do more than interpretation, advice, or confrontation. Ideally, as patients achieve small successes, they will be encouraged to venture forth into other areas. New and more age-appropriate sources of support and meaning can be established, leading to a more satisfying existence. During this process adolescents may even become aware of aspects of their upbringing that have led to the lack of preparedness for the demands of life.

Failures and rejections may be unavoidable, but it is the challenging task of the therapist to put such crises in perspective and to limit their effect from being generalized into a sense of total worth. Adolescents who are particularly socially inept generally benefit from an approach combining individual and group therapy. The latter can be used as a supplement to teach the basics of relationships with others. It is recommended that someone other than the individual therapist lead such groups, since much of the beneficial effect of individual therapy is the formation of an intimate, trusting alliance that is not shared with others. As youngsters begin to appreciate the mutual social impact of their peers, material resulting from interactions within the group is often discussed in individual sessions.

Introjective Depression

The clinical picture. Adolescents with introjective depression have little difficulty separating from their families and can function well independently. However, such adolescents carry within their psyches unrealistic internalizations of parental values that preclude any sense of psychological autonomy or satisfaction. They are wrought with guilt, self-criticism, and often suicidal ideation. They also exhibit a lack of responsiveness to their surroundings that is similar to that of adults with endogenous forms of melancholia. In contrast to the panic or agitation that colors anaclitic forms of depression, introjective depression is characterized by listlessness. Patients act as if they had given up on ever again enjoying life.

Hendin (1975) studied a group of such college students, each of whom had survived a suicide attempt. He reported that many denied themselves happiness or fulfillment because of irrational emotional ties to their parents. They could not participate in the more relaxed and pleasurable college atmosphere because an internalized sense of duty to their parents stifled any attempts at autonomous gratification. However, they also realized that by living out their parental commands, they were robbing themselves of a free and meaningful life. Suicide became an all too enticing solution to this inner conflict. The following clinical vignettes highlight these issues:

Case 1

A depressed adolescent presented with a sense of apathy, hypochondriacal concerns, and an increasing dislike for his studies, which he had formerly pursued avidly. This adolescent described himself as extremely close to his mother, who was chronically depressed. She, together with the patient, had formed an alliance against her spouse. She described her husband as coarse, uneducated, and vulgar, and appeared to despise him. She had decided early on that her son would not go into business as his father did, but would become a professional and enter a prestigious Ivy League college.

This ambition had been the boy's guiding principle ever since he could remember, and he had gladly accepted his favored role. However, as he entered his junior year of high school, he also wished to be accepted by his peers, who openly rebelled against school authorities and spent time drinking, playing pranks, and generally getting into mischief. Whenever he tried to be like his friends, he felt terribly guilty and worried that he was jeopardizing his future career. So he gradually withdrew from social activities, pretending to be more mature than his peers, but actually envying them. He spent more and more time alone, trying to excel in his studies even though they interested him less and less. Eventually, he lost his motivation for entering a superior college. Yet he could not bear the guilt associated with going to parties, dating, or just goofing off. In this context, he despaired of having anything to live for and developed gastrointestinal symptoms that absorbed his attention to the point that he was sure he had cancer and would soon die.

Case 2

A 15-year-old girl who had always excelled in school was seen after her grades dropped. She told her school guidance counselor that she saw no point in studying anymore, nor in doing anything, since life was pointless. For the preceding year this girl had been caught up in her parents' acrimonious divorce. She had gradually become her mother's protector and had slowly given up her own gratifying activities. Although her father had moved out, he made frequent calls to berate or threaten his wife. In an effort to put an end to the terror that these calls elicited in her mother, the patient began to intercept them. She tried to mollify her father in order to spare her mother and her siblings. She also became her mother's confidante and soon was the responsible adult in the household.

Because the girl was preoccupied with concern about her mother, she began to have difficulty concentrating. After school she neglected her friends and discontinued her activities so she could be home to censor possible calls from her father. Her feeling of responsibility was such that she felt guilty if she enjoyed herself with peers or even watched her favorite television programs. When doing so, she would see an image of her mother crying, and she would then reproach herself for her alleged selfishness. Eventually, her life was consumed by her parents' arguments and legal maneuvering and her mother's need for support. She had difficulty sleeping, lost weight, and constantly wondered about the purpose of life.

In therapy she spoke of a dream that she had during this period. In the dream she was at a public event with her mother and siblings. She saw her father in the crowded audience and was frightened that he would see them and make a scene. As he got closer to them, her dread increased. She told her family to leave, and, attempting to spare her mother possible torment, she went to her father. He then ordered her into his car with him and forced her to drive, despite her cries that she did not know how. The car raced forward, out of control, with her at the wheel. The police came and somehow stopped the car as she awoke.

This dream dramatically reflects her predicament; that is, by assuming her protector stance, she is forced into an adult role (driving) for which she is totally unprepared. She desperately needs outside help (the police) to put an end to it.

Therapeutic approaches.   Therapy with adolescents who have introjective depression should focus on identifying, examining, and modifying the irrational introjected values that are the cause of guilt and inhibition. Individual cases may vary substantially. Some adolescents may have assumed the responsibility for the happiness of a chronically depressed parent, while others may have developed fears that any deviation from familial expectations will result in abandonment by needed others. Still others may have strived to earn the acceptance of a demanding, overcritical parent whose values have been internalized. Another common situation is one in which parents have actually insisted on extreme behavior but by their own example have set up unrealistic models of conduct that conflict with the more hedonistic behaviors of adolescents. In all cases the therapist is seen as a more permissive and accepting parent who will support autonomy and satisfaction, and once a sense of trust is established, these patients often confess "secret" indiscretions. Positive responses to such revelations help to build a system of workable and logically based morals to replace the older tyrannical "shoulds" of childhood.

Depending on the severity of the symptoms, medication and/or hospitalization may be required. Most adolescents, however, experience a significant degree of symptomatic relief as soon as they unburden themselves to an empathic listener.

Summary

Both anaclitic and introjective depression are caused by an inability to successfully master the demands of adolescence. In both instances the illness can be traced back to a series of developmental failures that continue to impede growth into more mature modes of adaptation. Both have an insidious onset, with a variety of prior warning signs that are typically ignored. The actual precipitants are the new developmental demands that now lay bare this preexisting vulnerability. Treatment involves more than simply getting adolescents back on a normal developmental track. It involves facilitating a good deal of change in the way in which they perceive themselves and others, in how they create new goals for themselves and attempt to achieve these goals, and in the extent to which they allow themselves age-appropriate gratifications and pleasurable pursuits.

Bipolar Disorder

Although bipolar disorder is quite rare before puberty, it is not infrequent in adolescence. Stroeber and Carlson (1982) note that as many as 35% of all cases of manic-depressive illness begin during adolescence. It is thus essential that therapists be aware of the possibility of this disorder in severely depressed adolescents. Results from a follow-up study cited by the same authors indicate that bipolar outcome in severely depressed adolescents was significantly related to 1) the rapid onset of depressive symptoms, with psychomotor retardation and psychotic features; 2) strong family histories of mood disorder, including bipolar illness; and 3) hypomanic responses to administration of antidepressants.

As illustrated by the following case, the presentation of juvenile bipolar illness may show a puzzling prodromal course:

> A young woman seen in therapy had become withdrawn, anxious, and excessively dependent on her mother shortly after she reached puberty. Following a social disappointment several years later, she was hospitalized with acute delusional symptoms, panic, and confusion. Her symptoms cleared rapidly with neuroleptics, and she was discharged with a diagnosis of schizophreniform disorder. A while later, she started college. She became withdrawn and exquisitely sensitive to alleged snubs, and frequently demonstrated ideas of reference and quasiparanoid suspicion. By the end of her teenage years, this increasing social isolation had led to the emergence of a depression with some vegetative signs.
>
> When started on a low dose of a tricyclic antidepressant, she rapidly became agitated, euphoric, and argumentative. She began turning out paintings in quick succession and became impossible to get along with. At this point medications were discontinued and lithium carbonate was prescribed. This resulted in the remission of all symptoms. After this woman had reached therapeutic blood levels of lithium for some months, she stated that she felt normal for the first time since childhood.

This case is instructive because prior to having taken tricyclics there had been no evidence of mania.

Therapeutic Approaches

Psychotherapy for adolescents with bipolar illness is similar to that for adults with this disorder. Adolescents must learn to live with a chronic illness and understand the need for compliance with lithium maintenance. They must also improve upon any personality problems that arise either with or independently of their primary illness. Because their lives are so filled with change and emotional turmoil, these goals are extremely difficult to realize.

Some bipolar adolescents may discontinue medication impulsively, particularly if compliance interferes with social activities that are subject to peer pressure. Others may react to the need for maintenance medication as a further sign of inferiority or of being different from their peers. Still others may refuse to take medication.

As with any adolescent who requires continuous medication, youngsters with bipolar disorder must acknowledge that taking medication is their own responsibility and is not imposed upon them by others. The psychological meaning of taking medication and of having a chronic illness should be explored and discussed in a frank, open manner, with the expectation that patients will feel angry, cheated, and saddened at their fate. These understandable reactions become part of the psychotherapeutic process. They are best handled in an open, trusting situation where negative feelings can be neutralized and reconciled rather than acted out in a potentially destructive manner.

Summary

Psychotherapy of adolescents with mood disorders requires an appreciation of the particular vulnerabilities and strengths that are an inherent part of this developmental stage. Diagnosis may often be difficult because of the normal extremes of mood experienced by adolescents, as well as the frequent urgency and panic that confound the clinical picture. Therapy aims at helping youngsters meet the developmental tasks of adolescence in a satisfying manner, with the understanding that these individuals' are still in the process of growth and change. Ultimately, it is hoped that the honesty and openness of the therapeutic relationship will allow adolescents to discover genuine sources of meaning and gratification that will sustain them in the future.

References

Anthony EJ: Two contrasting types of adolescent depression and their treatment, in Depression and Human Existence. Edited by Anthony EJ, Benedek T. Boston, MA, Little Brown, 1975, pp 445–460

Arieti S: The psychotherapeutic approach to depression. Am J Psychother 16:397–406, 1962

Bibring E: The mechanism of depression, in Affective Disorders. Edited by Greenacre P. New York, International Universities Press, 1953

Blatt SJ: Levels of object representation in anaclitic and introjective depression. Psychoanal Study Child 29:107–158, 1974

Brown GW, Harris T: Social Origins of Depression. New York, Free Press, 1978

Csikszentmihalyi M, Larson R: Being Adolescent. New York, Basic Books, 1984

Easson WH: Depression in adolescence, in Adolescent Psychiatry, Vol 5. Edited by Feinstein SC, Giaovacchini P. New York, Jason Aronson, 1977, pp 257–275

Hendin H: Growing up dead: student suicide. Am J Psychother 29:327–338, 1975

Jacobson E: Adolescent moods and the remodeling of psychic structures in adolescence. Psychoanal Study Child 16:164–183, 1961

Leff ML, Roatch JF, Bunney WE: Environmental factors preceding the onset of severe depression. Psychiatry 33:293–311, 1970

Sandler J, Joffee WG: Notes on childhood depression. Int J Psychoanal 46:88–96, 1965

Stroeber M, Carlson G: Bipolar illness in adolescents with major depression. Arch Gen Psychiatry 39:549–555, 1982

Psychotherapy of Adolescents With Neurotic Disorders

JOHN E. MEEKS, M.D.

Chapter 10

Psychotherapy of Adolescents With Neurotic Disorders

*T*he nature of neurosis in adolescent patients may be somewhat less clear than it is in adults. However, the general characteristics of neurotic illness apply across age ranges.

First, adolescents with neurotic illnesses tend to internalize their problems just as neurotic adults do. Their conflicts are within themselves, their argumentative dialogues are internal, and their suffering is very personal. As a rule there is a felt sense of discomfort—either anxiety or depression, or a combination of the two—that is consciously and acutely experienced by the young person. Often these uncomfortable feelings are associated with negative attitudes toward the self and with self-blame. These patients feel that they have erred or are defective in some way and that these personal deficiencies cause the discomfort that they experience. At times they may blame others for some of their difficulties, but there is a discomfort in that position and the youngster is prepared, at least in a friendly atmosphere, to accept the responsibility for his or her own suffering.

At the same time that these youngsters are pained and self-derogatory, they retain a basic awareness that their concerns are not entirely rational and are not grounded in the objective universe around them. We say of these young people that their reality testing is intact. Indeed, they are often very aware that their concerns and apprehensions are unrealistic to the point of being "silly." This recognition does nothing to lower their discomfiture. Indeed, their recognition that their concerns are illusory merely makes them feel all the more foolish, weak, and "weird."

Neurotic symptomatology in adolescents may take protean form, often including episodes of overt anxiety, phobic defenses, obsessive behavior, compulsive preoccupations, and overt depression in various combinations. It is not unusual for symptomatology to be somewhat changeable, so the diagnosis should be based more on a careful overall assessment of the adolescents' functioning rather than on surface phenomenology alone.

It is important to clarify the relationship between psychological diagnostic thinking as presented in this chapter and the phenomenological nosology represented in DSM-III-R (American Psychiatric Association 1987). Levine (1961) suggested a six-level diagnostic approach in psychiatry, as follows:

1. Clinical (phenomenological) diagnosis
2. Dynamic diagnosis
3. Genetic diagnosis
4. Transference expectations
5. Countertransference expectations
6. Treatment possibilities

A psychological diagnosis such as "neurosis" is drawn from information and inferences related to the areas of dynamics and genetics. These observations will, of course, strongly guide transference and countertransference expectations. Taken together with the phenomenological diagnosis, psychological diagnosis also provides direction regarding treatment planning. The purpose of psychological diagnosis is to help the therapist to organize a conceptual picture of the patient's motivations, pattern of interpersonal interactions, and typical management of emotions.

The psychological structure discussed in this chapter might be found in some patients from a wide range of DSM-III-R diagnostic categories, including the anxiety disorders (separation anxiety disorder, avoidant disorder, and overanxious disorder), mood disorders (especially dysthymia), some identity disorders, some phobias and conversions, some adjustment disorders, and even in some youngsters who present primarily with disruptive behavior disorders.

The neurotic personality in adolescents is centered around a magical use of the imagination in an effort to resolve conflict within the patient. This general defensive patterning is to be contrasted with the adolescent who is more oriented toward "acting out" or the externalization of conflict. These externalizing youngsters attempt to resolve problems by changing the world around them rather than by creating internal fantasy structures. This distinction is not absolute, and, generally speaking, adolescents are more likely to externalize difficulties of any kind than are younger children or adults.

> Mick was a 13-year-old boy who developed a terror of attending school. He described himself as "a mama's boy" and worried that the examining psychiatrist would think him a "wimp." Hospitalized because his symptoms did not respond to outpatient therapy, he was panicky and eager to return home. He explained that he only made up the fear of school because he felt his parents favored his older brother, but then hastened to reassure the examiner, "Of course I love my brother."

This brief vignette clarifies the fact that although neurotic illnesses are "internal," they have a major communicative element and a major impact on the environment. In the interpersonal framework the neurotic illness can be seen as a demand or rebuke to others—especially family members—that the youngster cannot state directly. The symptom is an argument, but an argument that is subtle, indirect, apologetic, and self-wounding. The symptom also often has the effect of forcing a more intense and often more dependent connection with important others. This may be a more important source of "secondary gain" than is the superficially obvious avoidance of external anxiety-producing situations.

Personality Characteristics of the Neurotic Adolescent

The following points summarize in a descriptive way the presentation of these neurotic adolescents:

Negative self-esteem. This characteristic is frequently overt or fairly close to the surface. However, some youngsters, particularly those characterized by compulsiveness and overachievement, may be very reluctant to admit to their poor self-image.

Compliant, conventional, "people pleasing." These behaviors may be primarily superficial, with the patient's resentment and passive aggression reasonably apparent or even with quiet signs of open rebelliousness that are consciously disavowed:

> James, a 15-year-old boy with neurotic depression, followed the "letter of the law" scrupulously at his school. However, his clothes, though meeting dress code expectations, were always slightly unkempt and ragged. In a school where short, neat haircuts were the norm, James sported a tousled long mane. He was hurt and surprised when the assistant principal called him in and complained about his appearance.

Feelings of personal and physical deficiency. These feelings, especially those of smallness, weakness, and unattractiveness, often accompany neurotic behavior in adolescence. For example, later in therapy, James, the boy described above, attributed much of his difficulty to his short stature.

A professed sense of helplessness regarding symptoms. Often this is accompanied by adolescents disowning the problem as though it had fallen on them from the skies. At times neurotic adolescents profess themselves mystified and awed by their symptoms.

Preservation and clinging to symptoms. In spite of the fact that the symptoms are seen as ego-alien and outside of the patient's control, objective observation suggests that the patient is, in fact, clinging to his or her symptoms and preserving them.

For example, Mick, the 13-year-old with school avoidance described earlier, exclaimed at one point, "Maybe I don't want to grow up and take care of myself and be happy."

Overinvolvement of the family. The patient's family is usually somewhat anxious, concerned, and often overinvolved with the patient. For example, when attempting to discuss Mick's anxiety and difficulty in going to school, Mick's father would rather quickly slide into a pained tearfulness. It was obvious that he suffered his son's anxiety along with him.

Etiology of Neurotic Conflict in Adolescents

A neurotic illness represents a conflict between personal desire and the demands of socialization. As mentioned earlier this conflict has usually been largely internalized so that it is often expressed as a conflict between biological drives or their derivatives and the patient's superego.

This inner conflict may be latent in many relatively healthy adolescents and may never be expressed in actual clinical symptomatology. Indeed, some "neurotic" behaviors are commonly seen for periods of time during normal adolescence. Asceticism and compulsive preoccupation with some narrow element of life are common examples of the trend (A. Freud 1958). In most adolescents this neurotic behavior is time limited and does not in fact approach the severity that would interfere with development.

More serious neurotic conditions can be triggered by a variety of events (Meeks 1986b):

- Development itself may trigger neurotic conflict in the vulnerable adolescent. For example, Marie, a 14-year-old, was referred for treatment because of deteriorating school performance, social withdrawal, and preoccupation with philosophical and religious issues. Only 30 minutes into the initial interview Marie was giving an impassioned denunciation of the "boy craziness" of the other girls at her school. Marie's mother reported that her daughter had been frightened and angered by the onset of menses. In another case, Kay came to psychotherapy at the age of 15 because of tearfulness, insomnia, and somatic preoccupation. After several interviews she told her therapist that she found it difficult to sleep at night because she worried about her mother. She gradually connected this to fears that her father preferred her and, to her own shameful admission, that she felt superior—especially smarter and prettier—than her house-frau mother.
- Changes in living circumstances and family relationships may trigger conflict. Floyd, for example, at age 16, had to move to a different city when his father did not receive an expected promotion up the corporate ladder and was therefore given "banishment" to a different branch of the business. Floyd, always a happy-go-lucky, athletic, popular youngster, made an extremely poor adjustment to his new school and showed increasing irritability and withdrawal. He was referred for evaluation after very poor judgment had led him to minor legal difficulty.

Diagnostic evaluation revealed that Floyd's idealization of his father had been shattered by the business setback, an occurrence that gradually led to a disruption of his previous comfort with oedipal competition. He suddenly became quite frightened that he would surpass his father, thus leading to more shame and humiliation—an outcome that he unconsciously desired and consciously feared.

- Neurotic conflict can be triggered by specific events that tempt the youngster to forbidden behavior. This temptation may be toward unacceptable sexual behavior in response to seductiveness or unacceptable aggression in response to provocation. Mick, the patient described above, developed his school phobia when the family made a move to a new home in a new neighborhood. Mick loved his old neighborhood, had many friends there, and viewed his new home as isolated and "scary." However, he did not express any anger about the move to his family because he understood their wishes to make the change.

Within the general outline of neurotic illnesses that we have discussed, you will note that we have excluded the "traumatic neurosis," that is, the symptom pictures that would now be classified under post-traumatic stress disorder. We have also excluded those disorders that represent emergency efforts to utilize neurotic symptomatology to protect against psychotic disorganization. Perhaps the most common example is the frantic obsessive-compulsive behavior sometimes observed in the early stages of schizophrenic psychoses.

The illnesses that we will be discussing in this chapter might be illuminated further by considering two metaphors for their nature. The first metaphor is of the neurotic youngster as the victim of an evil curse. These youngsters often behave as though they have been told that they must behave as a frog rather than as a prince. In some cases one discovers that there is indeed a parental figure who knowingly or unknowingly acts to prevent the youngster from growing up and enjoying life. When the family dynamics are understood, a fear of the child's sexuality or competitive strength may be discovered, or a neurotic need on the part of the parent to maintain the child as somewhat helpless and overattached. In other cases the parent does not seem to be actually behaving this way but is perceived by the child as more restrictive than he or she actually is. In these cases the youngster may be more temperamentally driven to please or easier to influence, rather like the "easy child" described by Thomas et al. (1968). The following case illustrates this situation:

Doris, a 16-year-old sophomore, came into psychotherapy reluctantly because of friendlessness, preoccupation with school performance, and a general driven and frantic need for success at any cost. The family was mystified by her white-knuckle approach to life, since her older sister was relaxed, social, and rather happy-go-lucky. The mother felt that the two girls had shown a different temperamental style since birth, but she also noted that she had developed a medical illness when Doris was 3, which made her less available to provide dependency support for almost 2 years. In fact, during that time Doris was often warned by her sister and father not to bother her mother. Thus, it appeared that both temperamental and experiential factors led to Doris' development into adolescence as a person driven to complete self-sufficiency but to such an extreme degree that she elicited concern and attention from her family.

The second metaphor is of the emergency ramshackle shelter from which neurotic adolescents face life. They throw together this structure because they doubt the availability of proper supplies and equipment in the face of what they perceive to be major environmental dangers.

Both of these metaphors are pictorial ways of saying that neurotic illness is a compromise solution to a problem that results from either a misperception of the environment or the presence of caring and affectionate parents who for some reason find it difficult to tolerate genuine maturity and full emotional development in their child.

Confusing Diagnostic Presentations of Neurotic Conflict in Adolescents

As mentioned earlier the tendency of adolescents to express their concerns in actions directed toward the environment can lead to a presenting picture that seems more characterological than neurotic:

Marshall, a 17-year-old college freshman, came to therapy because of angry outbursts, excessive risk-taking behaviors such as driving too fast, and a reluctance to work in school. In the diagnostic interview he was angry, intimidating, and uncooperative. However, with his parents' support, Marshall was able to continue in therapy and to reveal major neurotic problems of social phobia, chronic depression, and work inhibition. Considerable work in therapy was necessary to help Marshall accept the idea that these symptoms were not a sign of weakness or of a lack of masculinity.

Many adolescents describe and experience their neurotic difficulties as though they were the direct and immediate result of parental behavior, as is shown in the following example:

> Kay, a 15-year-old adolescent discussed above, complained through the first 2 months of her psychotherapy that her mother restricted her excessively, treated her like a baby, and was interfering with Kay's wishes to find a boyfriend. However, as therapy progressed it became clear that Kay's own conflicts about sexuality and independence were the impediments to her movement into normal adolescence. As Kay began to work through some of her inhibitions, she became aware of her intense competitiveness with her mother and her tremendous anxiety about surpassing her.

Although Kay's mother did not play a major role in that youngster's difficulties aside from her impact as an internalized oedipal object, some parents do participate in the perpetuation of neurotic solutions. For example, Marshall, the 17-year-old college freshman described above, was supported in his avoidance of anxiety and eternal challenges by his overly invested and indulgent father.

Patient Selection for Outpatient Psychotherapy

The treatment of choice for almost all neurotic adolescent problems is outpatient psychotherapy, usually individual. Because the problems are primarily internalized, the dyadic relationship provides an opportunity for transference development, recognition of basic conflicts, and resolution of these conflicts within the therapeutic experience (Meeks 1986b). Group therapy is sometimes of value, particularly when symptoms involve social avoidance or stereotyped attitudes toward human relationships in a group setting (Kraft 1968). Although family therapy may be needed at times when ongoing family dysfunction is supportive of the neurotic conflict, it does not have as much application as in those instances where the family system pathology is still external and lived out in the day-to-day life at home (Minuchin 1974).

Dynamic individual psychotherapy requires a capacity to recognize feelings, verbalize them with reasonable honesty, and accept the anxiety that inevitably accompanies the exploration of an intense two-person interaction. Fortunately, most neurotic adolescents have this capacity, at least as a potential. The ability to observe the self and describe it with reasonable objectivity may be obscured early in the contact by the patient's focus on the symptoms. This extensive discussion of the symptoms may be necessary early in treatment in order to foster the development of a relationship because the patient expects sympathy and help in regard to his or her conscious suffering. The patient's parenthetical comments regarding his or her presumptions about the therapist's responses can be used to gradually lead to discussion and to a more direct emotional interaction.

> Diedre was a beautiful 16-year-old high school junior plagued by depression and low self-esteem. Her friends viewed her as superficial and flirtatious, for she was frightened to let anyone know her well. When her therapist commented that he did not think she would need an extended period of psychotherapy—intending that as a supportive comment—Diedre came to the next session distant and somewhat uncommunicative. When the therapist commented on her mood, the patient said, "I was thinking maybe I shouldn't come here anymore since you don't feel my problems are serious." Further discussion gradually revealed that Diedre felt the therapist was dismissing her unhappiness and loneliness as unimportant. The interview turned to Diedre's feelings that her older sister was more important than she within the family system.

Development of the Treatment Contract

Most neurotic patients are able to participate in the development of a mutually acceptable treatment contract. The exact form of the contract will vary from one patient to another, but in general outline it is an agreement that the patient's problems are the result of emotional conflict or confusion. The patient agrees to talk regularly with the therapist and to focus on his or her emotional concerns and human interactions during those talks. The family needs to have a similar understanding. The nature of the relationship between the therapist and the parents also should be discussed at the beginning of the treatment interaction. Most therapists feel that the patient's relationship with them should be confidential unless the patient's safety requires notifying the parents of some potential risk such as suicide or other dangerous behavior. Most parents are accepting of this rule if the reasons for it are explained and if they are assured that the therapist will maintain contact with them regarding progress of the treatment effort. Practical issues such as the location of the sessions, the fee, the frequency of therapy sessions, and the circumstances under which the parents and therapist will communicate should also be discussed at this time. Any questions or misunderstandings are important to cover as well, and it is wise to anticipate likely problems or difficulties, as the following case illustrates:

> Marshall, the phobic college freshman described above, was obviously going to be difficult to engage in a therapeutic alliance. In addition, the therapist anticipated that Marshall's father would be quick to support any resistance if Marshall presented the therapist as threatening or unsupportive in any way. Therefore, the therapist predicted that the beginning of treatment would be stormy and that Marshall would probably experience the therapist as insensitive and excessively confronting. The father was told sympathetically that the therapist realized that this would be extremely difficult to tolerate and that the father might wonder if the "cure was worse than the disease." The father was able to talk about his great sympathy for Marshall and the pain he experienced whenever Marshall suffered. This exchange proved very valuable in gaining the father's support for the treatment effort.

The Early Phases of Psychotherapy With a Neurotic Adolescent

The beginning psychotherapy sessions with neurotic adolescents tend to include various testing maneuvers that the adolescents undertake in order to deepen their understanding of the therapeutic relationship and to assure themselves that it will not merely be a repetition of earlier damaging interactions with important people in their life, as is seen in the following example:

> Tommie, a 17-year-old high school senior, came to treatment because of social isolation, general emotional inhibition, and mild anorexia. In early therapy sessions she was unusually forthright, warm, and spontaneous. She stated that it was a great relief to talk with someone to whom she could open up. She said, "I can be easy with you but not with someone that I could think of having sex with." The therapist replied, "Yes, it helps that I'm totally off limits." In a later session soon afterward, Tommie revealed with considerable shame and anxiety that at times she felt her father's physical and emotional treatment of her was excessively seductive and that she had witnessed him kiss a babysitter when she was 11.

Of course, many other potentially untherapeutic attitudes will also be checked for by the adolescent. Are you judgmental? Are you controlling? Do you intend to use the adolescent to demonstrate your own brilliance, power, or skill rather than being primarily motivated by the desire to be helpful? This list is endless, limited only by the adolescent's anxieties and the negative life experiences he or she has encountered.

Dealing with the potential unfairness of the therapist is only the neurotic adolescent's first task in utilizing psychotherapy. The second task is to develop an objective capacity for self-observation (Meeks 1986b). In many neurotic adolescents the initial effort to be self-descriptive is almost always self-critical. As mentioned earlier, the adolescent knows at some level that his or her symptomatology does not make logical sense. As a result the adolescent frequently belittles his or her illness as silly and unacceptable. The main instrument for changing this self-derision into objective self-reporting is the therapist's sympathetic but objective observation and commentary. The patient can gradually identify with the nonjudgmental yet honest attitude of the therapist. In addition, the therapist maintains a position that all of the patient's symptoms make sense once they are completely understood. It is at these times that the analogy of neurotic illness to a ramshackle emergency shelter can be helpful to the patient. The patient is told in essence, "You didn't just get up one morning and decide to have these uncomfortable ideas. Though you can't remember all of the reasons, the explanations are logical, and we will understand them better as we go along."

As the patient moves into a trusting relationship with the therapist, concerns are often awakened about the dependency gratification inherent in a positive relationship with an understanding adult. The relationship may stir anxieties around the possibility of becoming overly dependent or may make the patient more aware of dependency yearnings, thus creating shame and anxiety about possible "weakness." These concerns are best dealt with by recognizing them and noting their legitimacy in an adolescent who strongly desires greater independence. However, the focal nature of the dependency can be noted, and the relationship can be compared to other learning interactions voluntarily chosen by the patient— for example, working with a music instructor, athletic coach, or other person with particular skills that one needs to achieve a goal.

Many neurotic adolescents have an additional concern about their positive relationship with the therapist. They are concerned that they may be disloyal to one or both parents. This disloyalty relates not only to the attachment to the therapist but to angry or critical thoughts that may begin to arise in the open and exploratory dialogue that occurs in the psychotherapy setting. This issue of disloyalty is illustrated in the following example:

> Peter, a 14-year-old youngster referred for drug use and social isolation, was resistant to entering treatment and came only at his mother's insistence. After a few sessions, when Peter was beginning to warm up to the therapist, this reluctance was broached. Peter explained that it was his understanding that psychiatrists tend to "blame your problems on your parents" and that he did not want to hear such an idea. Eventually Peter needed to discuss his intense anger at his father, whose driven perfectionism and hypercritical attitude Peter had internalized as an extremely harsh superego.

Neurotic patients are also concerned that hidden conflicts will surface and that unacceptable ideas and feelings will be exposed to the therapist. This concern, of course, is quite legitimate. However, the adolescent does not usually experience the urge for expression of forbidden thoughts as originating from within. Instead, the therapist is often viewed as a tempter who will "try to make something out of" anything the patient says.

Modern teenagers are aware that the topics may concern sex, anger, sibling rivalry, and other issues that have been well publicized in the public press. Some patients may even intellectualize around these topics to avoid the possibility that they might appear unbidden in strong affective contexts.

> Sally, an extremely compulsive and inhibited 15-year-old with strong repression of her sexual drives, tended to be awkward and silent in early sessions. She stated that she had "nothing to talk about." After she gradually was able to discuss her thoughts and concerns around sexuality indirectly by discussing the dating behavior of her classmates, she began to relax. The discovery that the therapist was sympathetic and supportive while still recognizing the potential dangers of uncontrolled sexual behavior allowed Sally to gradually approach her own difficulties.

Transference in the Psychotherapy of the Neurotic Adolescent

It is obvious that the transference relationship is the key element in dynamic psychotherapy (Gitelson 1942). In the patient's distortions regarding the therapist, experienced with emotional intensity in the present, lies the opportunity for genuine restructuring of the personality. Distorted cognitions regarding the self and others occur in company with the painful affects that these cognitions occasion, all under the watchful eye of the therapist. This process allows these distortions to be corrected in a living relationship and, to some extent, to be understood in the light of the past. However, with the adolescent's drive toward progression and his or her future orientation, genetic reconstruction may be limited, even in intensive dynamic therapy.

Recognizing transference in adolescents is not always easy. Adolescents are less likely than adults to recognize the origin of distorted perceptions of the therapist as coming from themselves. Because of the tendency toward externalization and the incompletely developed cognitive skills that characterize the younger adolescent, adolescents often experience transference distortions as real and respond to them behaviorally. For example, the adolescent who views the therapist as threatening because of a hostile father transference may cower and whine in the sessions, sincerely believing that the therapist desires subservience. In one case, Tommie, the adolescent girl described above, first evidenced her developing oedipal transference by wearing baggy clothes to therapy sessions, leaving her hair unkempt, and complaining that she was gaining weight and becoming an "ugly fat pig."

Negative transferences are particularly problematic in the treatment of adolescents. Because the adolescent is less likely to realize the source of his or her discomfort than is the adult, negative transferences often lead to strong urges to terminate treatment. For example, Sally, the adolescent girl described above who was extremely uncomfortable regarding her sexual drives, experienced the therapist as critical and repressive. She demonstrated her ambivalence by wearing short skirts to the therapy session and then tugging downward on them. She told her mother that the therapist was grumpy and that she had nothing to say, and felt that therapy would not be helpful.

Many adolescents have negative transferences based on their own aggressivity and competitiveness. They anticipate rejection and retaliation from the therapist because of these wishes, as is seen in the following example:

> Claude, a 16-year-old depressed youngster, enjoyed baiting the therapist in a particular way. He would ask for advice and insist on converting any response into a suggestion. If he could not do so, he complained bitterly that the therapist never offered any good ideas. However, if he did find something he could consider a suggestion he would return in the next session or two to report rather gleefully that the suggestion did not work. During this same period of time he mentioned to his parents on more than one occasion that he did not think the therapist liked him.

A paradoxical response is often seen in psychotherapy with adolescents. The adolescent reaches a new depth of understanding, reveals important and very personal material in a session, and subsequently withdraws from the therapist and becomes less available. This sequence of events is most often related to these patients' difficulty with accepting the new insight about themselves and their tendency to project onto the therapist the critical and rejecting attitudes that in fact are theirs. In addition, therapy always includes a certain amount of negative response to the therapist related simply to the frustration of the patient's unrealistic hopes and wishes in regard to the therapist. In a very real sense we cannot avoid "letting our patients down."

As the patient develops transference reactions in the therapy process, the parents will react to these. The positive transference often occasions some envy and perhaps competitiveness from the parents, who often feel a sense of failure that they could not prevent or cure the neurotic illness in their child. If the original contract has been clearly presented and the therapist has carefully avoided parental roles such as deciding on family rules and limits, it is usually possible to help the family to recognize that the attachment to the therapist is focal and task related and does not represent a threat to the parental bond. Of course, it is important that this clarity regarding the relationship is maintained by the therapist. The psychotherapist can never replace the parenting figure in the real world, but from a countertransference point of view, competition with parents and a fantasied world of omnipotent and all-perfect parents are always a temptation.

When an adolescent is involved in a negative transference it often befalls the parents to maintain therapeutic contact in face of the adolescent's protest and wishes to terminate treatment. It is during these times that the therapist's alliance with the parents becomes so crucial. At these times the prior prediction of potential "rocky times" helps to support the parents' confidence that the therapist is competent when the patient is aggressively denying that possibility.

Countertransference

Countertransference reactions to adolescents are often intense and seem more likely to lead to acting out than do countertransference reactions toward adult patients. The intensity of emotion and the rawness of expression that characterize the adolescent increase the likelihood of strong personal responses. Countertransference reactions are usually unconscious although strong conscious attitudes toward the patient may be their surface manifestation. For example, dreading a therapy hour with a patient, strong feelings of boredom, and the like, alert the therapist to the possibility that something in the therapeutic interaction has activated unresolved problems in the therapist. Strong feelings of either optimism or pessimism about the outcome of treatment may also suggest countertransference. Any wish to move outside the parameters of the therapeutic relationship, thinking that would be more therapeutic than psychotherapeutic, is a red flag signaling countertransference.

Countertransference is a potentially constructive element in the therapeutic process. One might even argue that without some countertransference the therapy is so devoid of genuine empathy and intense feeling as to be somewhat lifeless. As a rule, when countertransference is recognized and its roots are pursued honestly by the therapist, the patient benefits. Although introspection and reflection may be valuable in sorting out countertransference responses, it is often necessary to have the objectivity of a listener in order to understand the response fully. Peer consultation with a colleague or even formal supervision is often indicted not only to benefit the patient but to allow for personal growth and ongoing self-discovery in the therapist.

Psychotherapeutic Process With the Neurotic Adolescent

As the initial storms of beginning psychotherapy are successfully weathered and transference and countertransference issues are subjected to therapeutic scrutiny, therapy settles into a steady working relationship. The sense of a therapeutic alliance can be felt in the cooperative atmosphere of the sessions and the virtually colleague-like relationship between the therapist and the patient. Indeed, during this period of treatment the identification with the therapist as therapist is so strong that a very high percentage of adolescents will express this psychological reality by voicing an ambition to become a psychotherapist themselves. They also identify with the objective, nonjudgmental, and supportive attitude of the therapist and often reveal it in their treatment of themselves and their friends and families. In addition, this positive tone in the relationship carries over to some interest in the therapist as a real person and a comfortable ability to utilize the therapist as an adult who can offer ideas and suggestions about the real world.

One important value of this aspect of the therapeutic process in neurotic patients is that it allows for a redefinition of interpersonal relationships. Generally speaking, neurotic adolescents feel that others are making unrealistic demands that these patients resent, while at the same time they distort their authentic nature in an effort to please others and gain their affection. The outcome is often that neurotic individuals are not well liked because their affection is not spontaneous and their efforts to make themselves agreeable are stereotyped and rigid rather than a response to the needs or wishes of others.

> Dave still had not had a real girlfriend by the time he was 17. He was extremely bitter about this because he saw other adolescent boys mistreat their girlfriends, argue with them, and get into trouble, while he was unfailingly polite, attentive, and generous to girls and never got into trouble. In the therapy relationship he demonstrated a similar "goody-two-shoes" behavior with the apparent expectation that the therapist would prefer him to all other patients. On one occasion the therapist was unavoidably detained and arrived late for a session with Dave. For the next 20 minutes Dave virtually bit his tongue in the process of insisting that the therapist's tardiness did not bother him in spite of the fact that he had very many important issues to discuss. He said, "I know you have things to do more important than talking with me." The therapist commented that Dave's behavior was making him uncomfortable and wondered if Dave had any negative reactions to his late arrival. Dave angrily denied any anger, but the discussion then turned to his annoyance with a girl who seemed to be withdrawing from him because she said he was "too serious." The therapist com-

mented sympathetically that even when Dave tried to do the things he felt people would like, it always seemed they wanted something else. At this, Dave's anger finally broke through. He exploded, "I don't want to be what you all want me to be—I want to be myself. There's nothing wrong with me as I am." The therapist agreed but wondered if there was some possibility for negotiation. The therapist told Dave that he felt badly about being late to the session because he knew that Dave was always punctual. At that point Dave was able to admit some "disappointment" that the therapist had been tardy.

The whole process of working through neurotic conflict and recognizing the many different forms and disguises that the conflict can take in day-to-day life occupies much of the time of the midpoint in psychotherapy. It should be recognized that during this process there will be fluctuations in the level of the therapeutic alliance partly caused by the very process of therapy itself and the vagaries of the transference–countertransference interactions. However, with the substrata of a basic therapeutic alliance, these variations are usually not powerfully disruptive and therapy can proceed on a reasonably steady basis.

Termination

Termination with the neurotic adolescent can occur when the patient's neurotic symptoms have sufficiently ameliorated to permit the young person to enter the mainstream of adolescent development and to become realistically involved with age mates and with his or her own family. Often the movement in this direction is quite clear and the time for termination is relatively easy to determine. However, with adolescent patients there are a few potentially confusing elements.

First, the fact that the adolescent, even free of neurotic difficulty, remains immature and in need of help and assistance may lead the therapist to change the therapeutic relationship into a long-term friendship. Although this is not altogether destructive, it may interfere with the patient's more appropriate efforts to get his or her needs met in relationships that involve more mutuality and opportunity for unrestricted intimate interaction.

A related problem comes up around the adolescent's acute sensitivity to adult rejection. It has been said with some truth that adolescents need to reject us and that they find it very difficult to tolerate us rejecting them. Unfortunately, for some adolescents, particularly the more dependent neurotic patients, the suggestion that it is time to terminate therapy may be experienced as a personal rejection. The adolescent may respond to this either by bolting prematurely from therapy without working through the leave-taking process or by increasing symptomatology in an effort to maintain the therapeutic relationship, as is shown in the following example:

> Tommie, the adolescent girl embroiled in oedipal conflict whom we have mentioned earlier, became extremely anxious around time for termination. Although she did not complain directly of termination, she behaved in such a way at home that the patient's mother called, questioning the decision and indeed wondering if her daughter wasn't just as ill as ever. A direct confrontation of the termination issues in the psychotherapy process quickly led to an amelioration of the exacerbation of symptoms.

Obviously, the process of termination is very important for adolescents, because it provides still another opportunity for them to learn that dependence can be voluntary, that it is not a matter of indefinite symbiosis, and that it can be utilized for the purpose of gaining mastery skills and a higher level of competence.

Of course it is not only the adolescent patient who must struggle with his or her strong feelings around termination. Termination can be extremely difficult for the therapist and often even more of a problem for the adolescent's parents. If the therapy has been successful and if the alliance between the therapist and the family has been constructive, the parents often feel that they are being bereft of a major support system; consequently, they may need considerable help in accepting the appropriateness of termination.

Termination of therapy with the neurotic adolescent does not mean that the adolescent will not or should not maintain future contact with the therapist. As mentioned earlier, there is a "real person" element to the relationship with an adolescent patient. Because of this the adolescent often wishes to keep the therapist apprised of his or her future achievements, and calls or visits to the therapist during holidays, vacations, times home from college or job, or other traditional occasions to "touch base" are common and constructive. It is also not unusual for the adolescent to propose at least once that therapy should begin again. This idea should be explored, but usually one discovers a situation of temporary stress that has reawakened the regressive urge for a dependent bond to the therapist. As a rule, a simple statement that the therapist understands the current difficulty the patient is having but does not believe that a resumption of therapy is indicated is a sufficient intervention.

References

Freud A: Adolescence. Psychoanal Study Child 13:255–278, 1958

Gitelson M: Direct psychotherapy of the adolescent. Am J Orthopsychiatry 12:1–14, 1942

Kraft IA: An overview of group therapy with adolescents. Int J Group Psychother 18:461–480, 1968

Levine M: Principles of psychiatric treatment, in The Impact of Freudian Psychiatry. Edited by Alexander F, Ross H. Chicago, IL, University of Chicago Press, 1961, pp 200–359

Meeks J: Diagnosis and psychotherapy of adolescents. Highland Highlights 10:2–6, 1986a

Meeks J: The Fragile Alliance, 3rd Edition. Melbourne, FL, Robert E. Krieger, 1986b

Minuchin S: Families and Family Therapy. Cambridge, MA, Harvard University Press, 1974

Thomas A, Chess S, Birch HG: Temperament and Behavior Disorders in Children. New York, New York University Press, 1968

Index